Analysis of
HEALTHCARE
Interventions That Change
Patient Trajectories

James H. Bigelow

Kateryna Fonkych

Constance Fung

Jason Wang

Sponsored by Cerner Corporation, General Electric, Hewlett-Packard, Johnson & Johnson, and Xerox

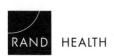

RAND HEALTH

The research described in this report was conducted within RAND Health and sponsored by a consortium of private companies, including Cerner Corporation, General Electric, Hewlett-Packard, Johnson & Johnson, and Xerox.

Library of Congress Cataloging-in-Publication Data

Analysis of healthcare interventions that change patient trajectories / James H. Bigelow ... [et al.].
   p. cm.
   "MG-408."
   Includes bibliographical references.
   ISBN 0-8330-3844-3 (pbk. : alk. paper)
   1. Health maintenance organization patients. I. Bigelow, J. H. (James H.) II. Rand Corporation.
   [DNLM: 1. Medical Informatics Applications. 2. Cost-Benefit Analysis. 3. Technology Assessment, Biomedical. W 26.5 A532 2005]

R729.5.H43A63 2005
362.1'068—dc22

2005022219

The RAND Corporation is a nonprofit research organization providing objective analysis and effective solutions that address the challenges facing the public and private sectors around the world. RAND's publications do not necessarily reflect the opinions of its research clients and sponsors.

RAND® is a registered trademark.

A profile of RAND Health, abstracts of its publications, and ordering information can be found on the RAND Health home page at www.rand.org/health.

Cover design by Barbara Angell Caslon

© Copyright 2005 RAND Corporation

Published 2005 by the RAND Corporation
1776 Main Street, P.O. Box 2138, Santa Monica, CA 90407-2138
1200 South Hayes Street, Arlington, VA 22202-5050
201 North Craig Street, Suite 202, Pittsburgh, PA 15213-1516
RAND URL: http://www.rand.org/
To order RAND documents or to obtain additional information, contact
Distribution Services: Telephone: (310) 451-7002;
Fax: (310) 451-6915; Email: order@rand.org

Preface

It is widely believed that broad adoption of Electronic Medical Record Systems (EMR-S) will lead to significant healthcare savings, reduce medical errors, and improve health, effectively transforming the U.S. healthcare system. Yet, adoption of EMR-S has been slow and appears to lag the effective application of information technology (IT) and related transformations seen in other industries, such as banking, retail, and telecommunications. In 2003, RAND Health, a division of the RAND Corporation, began a broad study to better understand the role and importance of EMR-S in improving health and reducing healthcare costs, and to help inform government actions that could maximize EMR-S benefits and increase its use.

This monograph provides the technical details and results of one component of that study. It examines interventions in the healthcare system that affect *patient trajectories,* i.e., the sequence of encounters a patient has with the healthcare system. The monograph analyzes interventions to improve patient safety, increase preventive services, expand chronic disease management, and foster healthier lifestyles. It estimates their effects on healthcare utilization, healthcare expenditures, and population health status.

Related documents are as follows:

- Richard Hillestad, James Bigelow, Anthony Bower, Federico Girosi, Robin Meili, Richard Scoville, and Roger Taylor, "Can Electronic Medical Record Systems Transform Healthcare? Potential Health Benefits, Savings, and Costs," *Health Affairs,* Vol. 24, No. 5, September 14, 2005.
- Roger Taylor, Anthony Bower, Federico Girosi, James Bigelow, Kateryna Fonkych, and Richard Hillestad, "Promoting Health Information Technology: Is There a Case for More-Aggressive Government Action?" *Health Affairs,* Vol. 24, No. 5, September 14, 2005.
- James Bigelow et al., "Technical Executive Summary in Support of 'Can Electronic Medical Record Systems Transform Healthcare?' and 'Promoting Health Information Technology'," *Health Affairs,* Web Exclusive, September 14, 2005.

- Kateryna Fonkych and Roger Taylor, *The State and Pattern of Health Information Technology,* Santa Monica, Calif.: RAND Corporation, MG-409-HLTH, 2005.
- Federico Girosi, Robin Meili, and Richard Scoville, *Extrapolating Evidence of Health Information Technology Savings and Costs,* Santa Monica, Calif.: RAND Corporation, MG-410-HLTH, 2005.
- Richard Scoville, Roger Taylor, Robin Meili, and Richard Hillestad, *How HIT Can Help: Process Change and the Benefits of Healthcare Information Technology,* Santa Monica, Calif.: RAND Corporation, TR-270-HLTH, 2005.
- Anthony G. Bower, *The Diffusion and Value of Healthcare Information Technology,* Santa Monica, Calif.: RAND Corporation, MG-272-HLTH, 2005.

The monograph should be of interest to healthcare IT professionals, other healthcare executives and researchers, and officials in the government responsible for health policy.

This research has been sponsored by a generous consortium of private companies: Cerner Corporation, General Electric, Hewlett-Packard, Johnson & Johnson, and Xerox. A steering group headed by Dr. David Lawrence, a retired CEO of Kaiser Permanente, provided review and guidance throughout the project. The right to publish any results was retained by RAND. The research was conducted in RAND Health, a division of the RAND Corporation. A profile of RAND Health, abstracts of its publications, and ordering information can be found at www.rand.org/health.

Contents

Figures

Tables

Summary

A *patient trajectory* is the sequence of events that involves the patient with the healthcare system. An intervention can affect trajectories by improving health, thereby reducing healthcare utilization or replacing a costly form of utilization (e.g., inpatient stays) with a more economical form of utilization (e.g., office visits to physicians or use of prescription medications). In this monograph, we examine the following selected interventions in the healthcare system that affect patient trajectories:[1]

- Implement Computerized Physician Order Entry (CPOE) as a means to reduce adverse drug events (ADEs) in both inpatient and ambulatory settings. ADE avoidance among inpatients reduces lengths of stay in the hospital. In an ambulatory setting, ADE avoidance may eliminate some hospital admissions and some office visits to physicians.
- Increase the provision of the following preventive services: influenza and pneumococcal vaccinations and screening for breast, cervical, and colorectal cancer. Vaccinations prevent some cases of influenza and pneumonia. Some people (mostly elderly) are hospitalized with these diseases. Screening identifies cancers earlier, improving survival and allowing less-extreme treatments to be employed.
- Enroll people with one of four chronic illnesses—asthma, chronic obstructive pulmonary disease (COPD), congestive heart failure (CHF), or diabetes—in disease management programs. Disease management reduces exacerbations of a chronic condition that can put the patient in the hospital.
- Persuade people to adopt healthy lifestyles and estimate the health outcomes if everyone did so: controlled their weight, stopped smoking, ate a healthy diet, exercised, and controlled their blood pressure and cholesterol as necessary with medications. Lifestyle changes can reduce the incidences (and ultimately the

---

[1] Not all interventions affect patient trajectories. For example, an intervention might replace manual transcription of physician notes by computerized voice recognition. This intervention and many others that do not affect patient trajectories are discussed in Girosi, Meili, and Scoville (2005).

prevalences) of a number of conditions that require substantial amounts of healthcare.

Because this work was part of a larger study, "Using Information Technology to Create a New Future in Healthcare: The RAND Health Information Technology (HIT) Project," we chose interventions that should be facilitated by HIT. HIT operates through several mechanisms. First, HIT can help identify the consumers eligible for the intervention by scanning an electronic database—for example, of medical records or claims data. Second, HIT can help consumers and providers adhere to "improved care" guidelines—for example, by reminding providers and patients when particular services are due and by providing instruction. Third, HIT may increase efficiency (e.g., using automation to reduce the need for home monitoring of patients by a nurse). Finally, HIT makes it easier to record and analyze the performance of an intervention, so that it can be improved over time. For example, one can use data collected on today's medical practices to develop still-better care guidelines.

Information technology is an *enabler*: It makes possible new ways of working (Hammer and Champy, 1993). But it does not guarantee that an enterprise will adopt new work processes, not in healthcare (Scoville et al., 2005) and not in other sectors of the economy (Bower, 2005). We have defined our interventions in terms of changes in the way the healthcare system works. Our results are therefore estimates of what *could* be, not predictions of what *will* be.

Estimating Potential Effects of Interventions

We estimated the potential effects of each intervention on healthcare utilization (e.g., hospital stays, office visits, prescription drug use), healthcare expenditures, and population health outcomes (workdays or schooldays missed, days spent sick in bed, and mortality). By *potential* we mean the maximum effect that could be achieved, assuming that everybody eligible to participate did so as effectively as possible. Although we do not expect the entire potential to be achieved, it provides an upper bound.

For each intervention, we first established baseline values for utilization, expenditures, and population health. For most interventions, our baseline was a database of patient trajectories developed from several years of the Medical Expenditure Panel Survey (MEPS), the third in a series of national probability surveys conducted by the Agency for Healthcare Research and Quality (AHRQ) on the financing and utilization of medical care in the United States. We created a database of patient trajectories (the sequences of events that involve patients with the healthcare system) from several years of the MEPS.[2] In addition to detailed information on healthcare utiliza-

---

[2] Files and documentation for each year are available at http://www.meps.ahrq.gov.

tion and expenditures, our database also includes data from the MEPS files that describe the patient, such as age, sex, ethnicity, health insurance status, measures of health status (e.g., self-reported health, days sick in bed), and medical conditions.

The MEPS data are particularly appropriate for estimating the effects of the above interventions, because the data link healthcare utilization, healthcare expenditures, and health outcomes in a single source. The consumer is the unit of observation. Each consumer uses healthcare services and pays for them (or they are paid for on his or her behalf), and each consumer reports health status information. There are sources that examine utilization alone, or expenditures alone, or population health status alone; the MEPS is the only publicly available, nationally representative source of data that puts them all together. The other sources are often considered more accurate within their specialized domains. Therefore, we compare MEPS with other sources and devise adjustments to align our MEPS-based estimates with them.

Next, we modified the baseline to reflect the presence of the intervention, basing our modifications on the published literature. We estimated the effects of the intervention to be the difference.

We performed a systematic review of both the peer-reviewed literature and the "gray" literature (i.e., HIT journals, conference proceedings, government reports, and healthcare trade journals) for studies that quantified the effects of our interventions. This review is described in Girosi, Meili, and Scoville (2005). We found a substantial number of articles that measured the effect of CPOE on adverse drug events and their costs. However, a handful of authors are responsible for the bulk of this research, so the data on effects are not nationally representative. Moreover, the ambulatory CPOE systems studied are mostly installed in hospital outpatient departments, not independent physicians' practices. Perforce, we extrapolated it to the national level anyway.

The data on preventive services come in two steps. First, there is a rich evidence base for the effects of preventive services on health. Second, there is much sparser literature on the effects of HIT on the performance of preventive services. Most of the latter articles report the effect of computer-generated reminders on the likelihood that physicians conform to guidelines, including guidelines related to preventive services.

We found many articles that estimated effects of disease management on healthcare costs and utilization, with a great deal of variation in the details of the interventions and the targeted population. HIT is generally considered to be an integral part of disease management, so there is no separate assessment of how much better disease management with HIT is than disease management without HIT.

We found quite a rich literature describing the effects of lifestyle changes on health. But we found few articles on the use of HIT to support lifestyle change. Our national efforts to influence lifestyles have mostly taken the form of public health campaigns, such as the campaigns to reduce tobacco use and to improve nutrition. In the absence of data, we are forced to argue that it is plausible that HIT can play a role in lifestyle change.

The Evolution of Intervention Effects Over Time

We have estimated the effects our interventions would have in the healthcare system of the year 2000. In essence, we imagined that somebody changed the healthcare system back in, say, 1980, and that the data collected by MEPS in 1996–2000 (the data we used to construct our trajectory database) would have been different. It is this difference that we attempt to estimate.

In reality, of course, these interventions would be implemented in the present, and their effects would occur years in the future. We devised adjustments for future demographic changes to the year 2020, and we could, if we wished, adjust expenditure effects for assumed increases in healthcare costs. But these adjustments tell us nothing new about the interventions. For example, if we estimate that an intervention would reduce the expenditures captured in the 2000 MEPS data by 15 percent, our estimates adjusted for demography and inflation show a reduction little different from 15 percent.

We chose not to speculate about other possible changes to the healthcare system. For example, technological changes will flow from genomics, nanotechnology, and stem-cell research. Cultural attitudes may change—for example, about whether basic healthcare is a right and possibly about how much end-of-life care one is entitled to. And the healthcare system could respond to the changes wrought by our interventions in different ways (e.g., if hospital stays for today's reasons decline, either hospitals could be closed or the system could find other reasons to treat people in hospital). An investigation of these factors was far beyond the scope of the present project.

Potential Effects of the Interventions

Next, we describe how we estimated the potential effects of the interventions listed earlier. Recall that by *potential* we mean the maximum effect that could be achieved, assuming that everybody eligible to participate did so as effectively as possible. Although we do not expect the entire potential to be achieved, it provides an upper bound.

Preventing Adverse Drug Events in the Inpatient Setting

Evidence suggests that Computerized Physician Order Entry can be effective in both hospital and ambulatory environments. We examined the potential effects of using CPOE in both environments as a means of reducing adverse drug events.

To estimate the effects of inpatient CPOE for the nation as a whole, we took an overall rate of ADEs per patient-day from the literature, and we distributed it to hospital stays with diagnoses that a physician identified for us as being most likely to be associated with ADEs. Descriptions of hospital stays (including diagnoses and an identification of the hospital hosting the stay) came from the Nationwide Inpatient Sample (NIS), a public-use file available from AHRQ's Healthcare Cost and Utilization Project (HCUP).[3] Hospital characteristics came from the American Hospital Association (AHA) annual survey of the nation's hospitals.[4]

Figure S.1 shows the results of installing CPOE only in large hospitals, where we have varied the dividing line between large and small hospitals. We look at ADE avoided and at bed-days and dollars saved. Clearly, most of the effects can be realized by installing CPOE only in hospitals with at least, say, 100 beds. But it is not enough to install CPOE only in the really large hospitals.

These effects are not large. The total savings of $1 billion compares with total expenditures on hospital care of $413 billion in 2000.[5] A hospital with over 500 beds will save about $1 million per year, according to this analysis. Smaller hospitals save less, and, indeed, save somewhat less per bed.

Figure S.1 also splits the benefits according to whether the patient is under 65 years of age or 65 and older, as an approximation of the Medicare population. Only about 13 percent of the population is 65 or older, but it accounts for more than its proportional share of hospital utilization (37 percent of hospital stays and 48 percent of hospital bed-days). But we calculated that about 62 percent of the benefits of inpatient CPOE would accrue to patients in the older group, because a higher fraction of patients 65 years and older have diagnoses associated with ADEs.

---

[3] Agency for Healthcare Research and Quality (AHRQ), Rockville, Md. Available at http://www.ahcpr.gov/data/hcup.

[4] The *AHA Annual Survey Database* may be purchased from the AHA at www.ahaonlinestore.com.

[5] National Health Expenditures are available at www.cms.hhs.gov/statistics/nhe. As of this writing, estimates are available for the years 1960 through 2002. Projected expenditures are available from 2003 through 2013.

Figure S.1
Annual National-Level Effects of Using CPOE to Avoid Inpatient ADEs, by Hospital Size

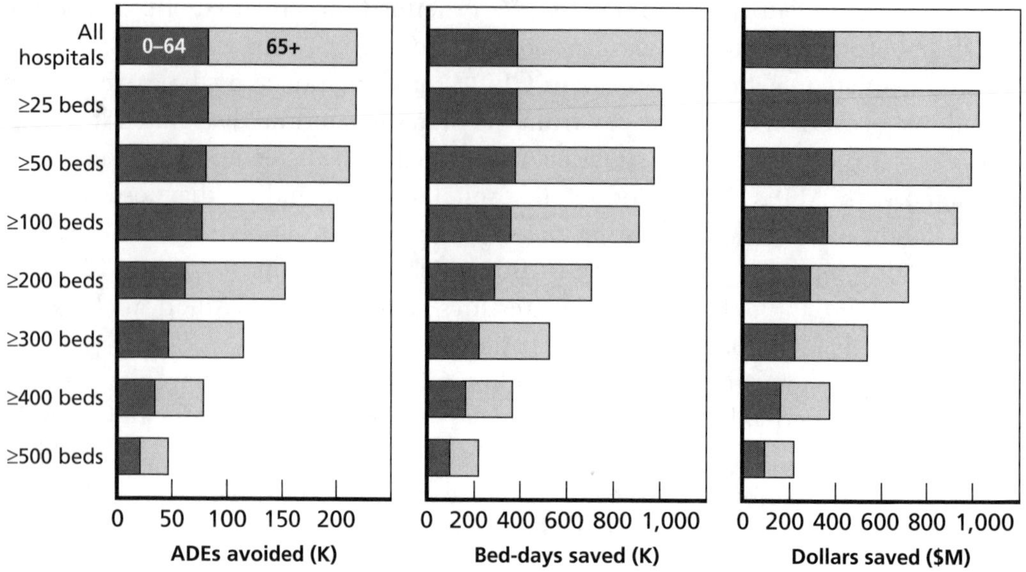

Preventing Adverse Drug Events in the Ambulatory Setting

We used a similar process to estimate the implications of ambulatory CPOE for the nation. Again, we took from the literature an overall rate for ADEs per visit to a physician's office, and we distributed them to visits where problem drugs (i.e., the drugs most likely to be involved in ADEs) were prescribed. Descriptions of office visits came from the National Ambulatory Medical Care Survey (NAMCS) (National Center for Health Statistics, multiple years).

Figure S.2 shows the results of installing CPOE, by practice size and ownership, which one might view as a proxy for financial strength. National savings from avoiding outpatient ADEs are around $3.5 billion. Savings from substituting generic drugs for brand-name drugs (typically accomplished by urging physicians to choose drugs from a formulary) exceed $20 billion per year.

Unlike with hospital-based CPOE, one should not ignore the small players when considering physicians' offices. About 37 percent of the potential savings comes from solo practitioners. The question is, Can single practitioners afford ambulatory CPOE? Also, some group practices will have only two or three physicians, and they, too, may have trouble affording ambulatory CPOE.

Figure S.2
Annual National-Level Effects of Implementing Ambulatory CPOE in Physicians' Offices

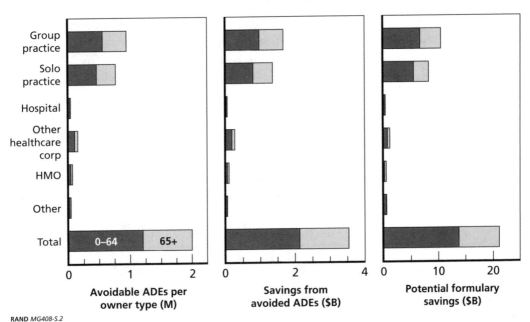

RAND *MG408-S.2*

Patients 65 years and older account for about 40 percent of ADEs, but for only 35 percent of the savings that comes from prescribing cheaper drugs. An office visit by a person 65 or older is more likely to be associated with an ADE than is a visit by a person under 65, probably because the elderly take more drugs on average.

Not shown in the figure are potential savings of $6.4 billion per year by eliminating duplicate laboratory tests and diagnostic radiological procedures. These savings will accrue to practices only if they are associated with capitated patients.[6] Otherwise, the savings accrue to the payer and (one hopes) will eventually be passed along to society as a whole in the form of lower health insurance premiums.

Vaccination and Disease Screening

Reminders provided by Electronic Medical Record Systems have been shown to increase the likelihood that patients receive influenza and pneumococcal vaccinations, and screening for breast cancer, cervical cancer, and colorectal cancer.

To estimate the effects of these preventive interventions, for each condition to be prevented, we selected the population from our MEPS analysis file that the United States Preventive Services Task Force (USPSTF) recommends should receive the intervention. For example, the USPSTF recommends that everybody 65 and over

---

[6] Under a capitation arrangement, a physicians' group agrees to provide all necessary care for a fixed payment per covered person. A more usual arrangement, called fee for service, pays the physician for each service rendered.

should receive an influenza vaccination each year. Therefore, to model flu vaccination, we selected all MEPS respondents of age 65 or older.[7] We combined these data with information from the published literature on the fraction of people that currently receives the service, and costs and benefits per instance of the service.

Table S.1 shows our estimates of some of the effects of these five preventive services. These estimates assume that the services are rendered to 100 percent of people not currently complying with the USPSTF recommendation. We made optimistic assumptions regarding the health benefit estimates as well. We concluded

Table S.1
Summary Results for Five Preventive Services (assumes 100-percent participation)

	Influenza Vaccination	Pneumococcal Vaccination	Screening for Breast Cancer	Screening for Cervical Cancer	Screening for Colorectal Cancer
Program Description					
Target Population	65 and older	65 and older	Women 40 and older	Women 18–64	50 and older
Frequency	1/yr	1/lifetime	0.5–1/yr	0.33–1/yr	0.1–0.2/yr
Population Not Currently Compliant	13.2 M	17.4 M backlog; 2.1 M new persons/yr	18.9 M	13 M	52 M
Financial Impacts					
Program Cost (with 100% compliance)	$134 M to $327 M/yr	$90 M/yr	$1,000 M to $3,000 M/yr	$152 M to $456 M/yr	$1,700 M to $7,200 M/yr
Financial Benefits	$32 M to $72 M/yr	$500 M to $1,000 M/yr	$0 to $643 M/yr	$52 M to $160 M/yr	$1,160 M to $1,770 M/yr
Health Benefits					
Reduced Workdays Missed	180,000 to 325,000/yr	100,000 to 200,000/yr			
Reduced Days Abed	1.0 M to 1.8 M/yr	1.5 M to 3.0 M/yr			
Deaths Avoided	5,200 to 11,700/yr	15,000 to 27,000/yr	2,200 to 6,600/yr	533/yr	17,000 to 38,000/yr
Years of Life Gained				13,000/yr	138,000/yr

---

[7] The USPSTF recommends vaccination for persons in certain high-risk groups as well, but we do not attempt to identify those persons in the MEPS database.

that all these measures provide health benefits, and all except pneumococcal vaccination increase healthcare utilization and expenditures. Pneumococcal vaccination is an exception, because only one dose is needed after age 65, and it continues to provide protection for life.

Chronic Disease Management

Effective disease management requires that the provider maintain a patient registry, and that enrolled patients have the means to receive advice and support from the provider and to send current symptoms and questions to the provider, all in real-time. These functions are best performed by information technology.

To estimate the costs and benefits of enrolling people with chronic illnesses in disease management programs, we examined management programs for four conditions: asthma, chronic obstructive pulmonary disease, diabetes, and congestive heart failure. For each condition, a disease management program seeks to avoid costly hospitalizations and visits to the hospital emergency department. For these encounters with the healthcare system, the program substitutes regular contacts with a provider (sometimes telephone calls with a nurse case manager, sometimes group or individual visits with a physician). Often, patients in a disease management program use more medications than those not in such a program. All of these changes occur in the short term—i.e., within a year or so of the patient enrolling in the program.

Figure S.3 shows the results we obtained, assuming that 100 percent of the people eligible for each disease management program participated. We also assumed that, in the analysis database (our baseline), nobody participated in programs to manage these diseases. On both counts, our results are optimistic. These programs reduce hospital utilization substantially, at the cost of increased office visits to physicians and an increase in the use of prescription drugs. However, there is a potential net savings of several tens of billions of dollars. Keeping people out of the hospital is, of course, a health benefit, but we also expect reductions in days lost from school and work, and days spent sick in bed. The reductions in days shown in the figure are optimistic, because some days lost or sick will be for reasons unrelated to the condition being managed.

Effects of Lifestyle Change

A program of lifestyle change would have huge benefits if everybody controlled their weight, stopped smoking, ate a healthy diet, exercised, and controlled their blood pressure and cholesterol as necessary with medications. In the long run, the population would be much healthier, and it would use substantially less healthcare. But for these outcomes to happen, consumers must come to see themselves as their own front-line caregivers. They need the information, the skills, and the confidence

Figure S.3
Annual Effects of Four Disease Management Programs (assumes 100-percent participation)

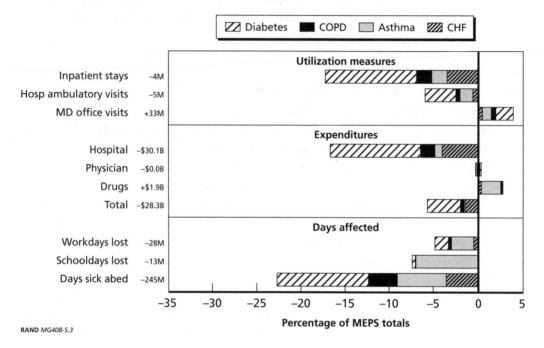

RAND *MG408-S.3*

to keep themselves healthy to the degree that they can, and to seek help when events slip out of their control. By itself, information technology will not bring about this transformation. But we argue that the transformation cannot happen without information technology.

We modeled the effects of a program of lifestyle change by changing the incidence of selected chronic medical conditions. Smoking cessation can reduce the incidence of COPD and smoking-related cancers. Combinations of diet, exercise, weight control, and medications can control hypertension and hyperlipidemia, which are risk factors for more serious cardiovascular conditions. Weight control can reduce the incidence of diabetes and its complications. For our example, we assumed that lifestyle changes can reduce the incidence of each condition to 40 percent of its current level. Over the long term, this reduction in incidence will result in a reduction in *prevalence*—the number of cases in the population at a point in time.

Figure S.4 shows the results. Again, we assumed that 100 percent of the population participates in the program. But if, by some wizardry, that participation could be achieved, there would be huge benefits. The total expenditures captured in the MEPS file declined by over 20 percent.

Figure S.4
Annual Effects of Lifestyle Changes (assumes 100-percent participation)

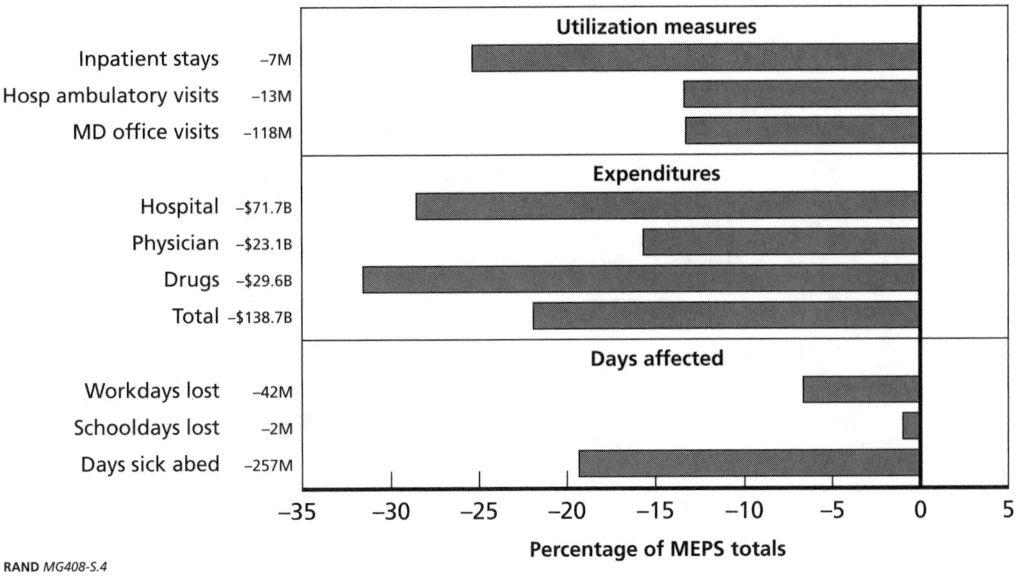

RAND *MG408-S.4*

Combining Disease-Management and Lifestyle-Change Effects

To combine effects of disease management with those of lifestyle change, we cannot simply add the two estimates. In the long term, lifestyle change reduces the number of people with chronic diseases. Thus, fewer people are eligible for disease management programs. Figure S.5 shows the results. As expected, the combined results are smaller than the sum of the individual results. The sum of expenditure reductions from Figures S.3 and S.4 is $167.0 billion; the combined reduction is "only" $146.9 billion.

Realistic Participation Rates

To obtain the results in Figures S.3, S.4, and S.5, we made the unrealistic assumption that 100 percent of those eligible participated in each intervention. To obtain a more realistic estimate, we scale participation down to 50-percent participation in our four disease-management programs and 20-percent participation in a program to foster healthier lifestyles. Experience shows that patients comply with medication regimes about 50 percent of the time on average, although there is a great deal of variation from one study to another. Studies show that patients comply with

Figure S.5
Combined Effects of Disease Management Plus Lifestyle Change (assumes 100-percent participation)

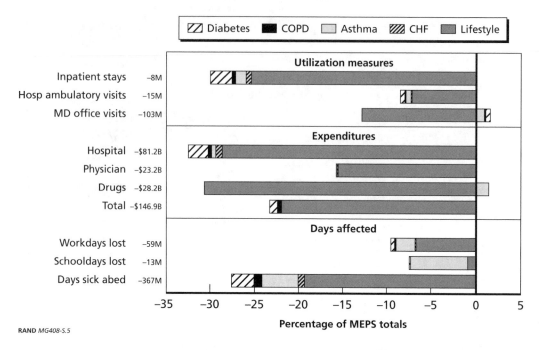

RAND *MG408-S.5*

their physicians' lifestyle recommendations only about 10 percent of the time (Roter et al., 1998; Haynes, McDonald, and Garg, 2002). Optimistically, we double that figure.

Figure S.6 shows the benefits realized if we apply these participation rates. Our estimate of total monetary savings is only about 30 percent that of the 100-percent-participation case, and other benefits drop by similar proportions. Clearly, there are large potential benefits that will not be realized by a "business as usual" approach to healthcare.

Increasing Consumer Participation

What may be the most profound aspect of the HIT-mediated transformation of healthcare is requiring much more from the patient (or consumer, since a person does not have to be sick to receive health care) than traditional health care does. Through disease management and lifestyle changes, healthcare ceases to be a commodity that healthcare providers deliver to passively accepting patients. Instead, it becomes an activity in which consumers and providers engage jointly and cooperatively. Think of the analogy of a coach and a player. The coach provides technical knowledge, advice, support, and encouragement to the player. But,

Figure S.6
Combined Effects of Disease Management and Lifestyle Change
(assumes 50-percent disease management and 20-percent lifestyle participation)

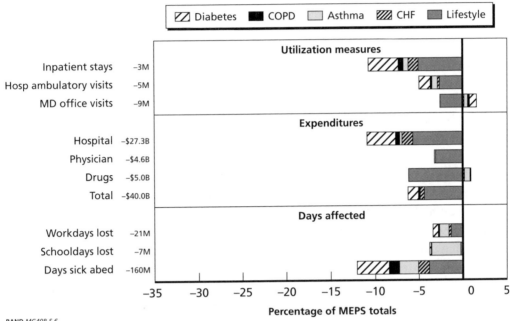

RAND *MG408-S.6*

ultimately, the player is the one who scores the points. Similarly, the healthcare provider has the technical knowledge. But especially for chronic care and lifestyle change, if the patient doesn't do it, it doesn't get done.

There can be no coaching without communication. Similarly, to help consumers become effective self-caregivers, they must be connected to the people who will coach them. They must have access to the appropriate knowledge, and they must have opportunities to learn needed skills. They must have a number to call when they need advice or encouragement. In short, consumers, information sources, and providers must all be connected via a community network.

Connecting the community is necessary but not sufficient. Much needs to be learned about how to increase consumers' participation in their own care. The quality and quantity of participation need to be measured routinely and subjected to systematic improvement efforts. Nonparticipants need to be identified and ways found to overcome individual barriers to participation and to promote convenient and pleasant ways to maintain and improve everyone's health.

We do not have evidence to tell us how well such a process can work, or how long it may take. But there is evidence that people adopt healthier behaviors when they understand the reasons and they have the incentive. For example, the anti-smoking campaign has reduced the fraction of people over 18 that smokes from 42 percent in 1965 to 23 percent in 2001 (National Center for Health Statistics,

2003)—a 45-percent reduction. It has done so, in part, by making smoking more expensive and, in part, by making it less acceptable. Twenty years ago, almost nobody objected to smokers lighting up in their homes or offices. Today, almost nobody—in California, at least—would fail to object.

Realizing the Potential

We estimated the *potential* benefits of our interventions, meaning the maximum effect that could be achieved, assuming that everything goes as well as it possibly could. But the benefits actually realized will generally be less than the potential benefits we have estimated—and, perhaps, much less. A major reason is that our interventions require that the healthcare system undergo some change. Change is disruptive, and people resist it. But unless providers, payers, and consumers do change, the benefits will not be realized.

Most existing HIT applications operate within a single provider organization, and they require changes of only the staff of that organization. Even within a single organization, those changes are not made easily; the staff must experiment to learn how to take advantage of HIT. Among our interventions, this is true of inpatient CPOE, and of ambulatory CPOE, which is installed in a hospital outpatient department, and which has access to ancillary services (e.g., pharmacy, laboratory, and radiology) provided by the hospital.

But some interventions require coordination among providers in different organizations. An Electronic Medical Record (EMR) installed in a physician's office has much greater potential value if it connects to other providers and, for that matter, to the consumer. If it connects to the pharmacy, for example, much the same opportunities to intercept medication errors and ADEs are enabled that an inpatient EMR offers. If it connects to the consumer, both physician and consumer can be reminded when preventive services are due.

Our remaining interventions require that the consumer be made into an expert provider of his or her own care, rather than a passive recipient. This is the change discussed in Chapter Eight. There, we point out that the consumer is already an active participant, but that the healthcare system rarely helps the consumer to participate expertly. Disease management requires both coordination of multiple providers and expert participation by the patient. But the chronically ill patient has an immediate incentive to learn how to manage his or her symptoms. Patients do not, after all, go to the emergency room (ER) for the pleasure and excitement it affords. Lifestyle change requires expert participation by the patient, but without the obvious immediate incentive.

Our interventions, their potential benefits, and the relative risk of realizing that potential are summarized in Table S.2. The relative risk is our own subjective assessment of how difficult it is likely to be to realize a large fraction of the potential benefit. It is based partly on the strength of the evidence and the amount of experience, and partly on the amount of change our interventions require of the healthcare system.

For each of our interventions, there is some risk that the potential benefits will not be fully realized, and, as we move down the rows of Table S.2, the risk becomes greater. But we need not leave the matter entirely to chance. Taylor et al. (2005) discuss policies that we think could speed up adoption of HIT; facilitate the development of the networks needed to connect and coordinate payers, providers, and consumers; and promote efforts to monitor compliance with prevention and disease management guidelines; and to measure and improve healthcare quality. Monitoring and measurement are important for all our interventions, but especially for programs to promote lifestyle change. Because we know least about how to promote such changes, the greatest amount of experimentation will be required to get this aspect right.

Table S.2
Summary Potential Net Benefits of Interventions

Class of Intervention	Monetary Net Benefits (billion)	Relative Health Benefits	Relative Risk
CPOE, inpatient	$1.1	Modest	Low
USPSTF-recommended preventive services	Break-even or small net cost	Modest	Medium
CPOE, ambulatory	$31.2	Modest	Medium
Disease management with 100% participation (diabetes, CHF, asthma, and COPD)	$28.3	Large	High
Lifestyle change with 100% participation	$138.7	Very large	Very High

Acknowledgments

We benefited greatly from the counsel of several RAND colleagues. We had numerous discussions with Robin Meili. Matthias Schonlau advised us on statistical matters. Scott Ashwood provided statistical programming help.

The monograph was much improved by the thoughtful comments of our two reviewers, Joel W. Cohen, Ph.D., of the Agency for Healthcare Research and Quality (AHRQ) and Emmett B. Keeler, Ph.D., of RAND. Marian Branch skillfully edited the manuscript.

Acronyms

ACE	anglotensin-converting enzyme
ACPOE	Ambulatory Computerized Physician Order Entry
ACS	American Cancer Society
ADE	adverse drug event
ADL	activities of daily living
ADR	Adverse Drug Reaction
AHA	American Hospital Association, American Heart Association
AHRQ	Agency for Healthcare Research and Quality
AMA	American Medical Association
AMI	acute myocardial infarction
AOA	American Osteopathic Association
BMI	body mass index
BP	blood pressure
CAD	coronary artery disease
CCC	Clinical Classification Code
CCM	Chronic Care Model
CD	compact disc
CDC	Centers for Disease Control and Prevention
CF	cystic fibrosis
CFAH	Center for the Advancement of Health
CHF	congestive heart failure
CITL	Center for Information Technology Leadership
CMS	Centers for Medicare and Medicaid Services
COPD	chronic obstructive pulmonary disease

CPOE	Computerized Physician Order Entry
DHHS	Department of Health and Human Services
DMAA	Disease Management Association of America
EC97	*1997 Economic Census*
ED	emergency department
EMR	Electronic Medical Record
EMR-S	Electronic Medical Record System
ER	emergency room
FDA	Food and Drug Administration
FOBT	fecal occult blood test
GOLD	Global Initiative for Chronic Obstructive Lung Disease
HbA1c	glycosylated hemoglobin
HCRIS	Healthcare Cost and Reporting Information System
HCUP	Healthcare Cost and Utilization Project
HIT	Health Information Technology
HIV	human immunodeficiency virus
HMO	health maintenance organization
IADL	instrumental activities of daily living
ICD-9	*International Classification of Diseases,* Revision 9
IHI	Institute for Healthcare Improvement
IOM	Institute of Medicine
IT	information technology
MCBS	Medicare Current Beneficiary Survey
MD	Medical Doctor
MEPS	Medical Expenditure Panel Survey
MRI	magnetic resonance imaging
MSA	Metropolitan Statistical Area
NAICS	North American Industrial Classification System
NAMCS	National Ambulatory Medical Care Survey
NCHS	National Center for Health Statistics
NEC	not elsewhere considered
NHA	National Health Accounts

NHAMCS	National Hospital Ambulatory Medical Care Survey
NHE	National Health Expenditures
NHIS	National Health Information Survey
NHLBI	National Heart, Lung, and Blood Institute
NIAID	National Institute of Allergies and Infectious Diseases
NIDDK	National Institute of Diabetes and Digestive and Kidney Diseases
NIH	National Institutes of Health
NIS	Nationwide Inpatient Sample
NNHS	National Nursing Home Survey
NOS	not otherwise specified
NPC	National Pharmaceutical Council
NYHA	New York Heart Association
OACT	Office of the Actuary (within CMS)
P&CS	physician and clinical services
PAP	*Papanicolaou*
PCP	primary care physician
RL	revenue line
SAS	Service Annual Survey, Statistical Analysis System
SE	standard error
SQL	structured query language
USP	United States Pharmacopeia
USPSTF	United States Preventive Services Task Force
VA	Veterans Administration
WHO	World Health Organization

CHAPTER ONE

Introduction

James H. Bigelow, Ph.D.

A *patient trajectory* is the sequence of events that involves the patient with the healthcare system. As part of a larger study, "Using Information Technology to Create a New Future in Healthcare: The RAND Health Information Technology (HIT) Project," we examined selected interventions in the healthcare system that affect patient trajectories and that should be facilitated by HIT.[1] We have identified four classes of trajectory-changing interventions and we have selected some important interventions in each class:

- Implement Computerized Physician Order Entry (CPOE) as a means to reduce adverse drug events (ADEs).
- Increase the provision of the following preventive services: influenza and pneumococcal vaccinations and screening for breast, cervical, and colorectal cancer.
- Enroll people with one of four chronic illnesses—asthma, chronic obstructive pulmonary disease (COPD), congestive heart failure (CHF), or diabetes—in disease management programs.
- Persuade people to adopt healthy lifestyles and estimate the health outcomes if everyone did so: controlled their weight, stopped smoking, ate a healthy diet, exercised, and controlled their blood pressure and cholesterol as necessary with medications.

We estimated the effects of each intervention on healthcare utilization (e.g., hospital stays, office visits, prescription drug use), healthcare expenditures, and population health outcomes (workdays or schooldays missed, days spent sick in bed, mortality). These interventions generally affect trajectories by improving health and thereby reducing healthcare utilization, or by reducing a costly form of utilization

---

[1] Not all interventions affect patient trajectories. For example, an intervention might replace manual transcription of physician notes by computerized voice recognition. This intervention and many others that do not affect patient trajectories are discussed in Girosi, Meili, and Scoville (2005).

(e.g., inpatient stays) and increasing a more economical form (e.g., office visits to physicians, or prescription medications). For example,

- ADE avoidance among inpatients reduces lengths of stays in the hospital. In an ambulatory setting, ADE avoidance may eliminate some hospital admissions and some office visits to physicians.
- Vaccinations prevent some cases of influenza (flu vaccination) and pneumonia (pneumococcal vaccination). Some people, especially the elderly, are hospitalized with these diseases.
- Disease management is intended to reduce exacerbations of a chronic condition (asthma, congestive heart failure) that can put the patient in the hospital.
- Lifestyle changes can reduce the incidences (and ultimately the prevalences) of a number of conditions that consume substantial amounts of healthcare.

In general, HIT is known to facilitate these interventions in three ways. First, HIT can help identify the consumers eligible for the intervention. The provider of a disease management program, for example, can identify patients with the target disease by scanning an electronic database of medical records (if a physician operates the program) or claims data (if a payer operates the program). Second, HIT can help consumers and providers adhere to "improved care" guidelines—for example, by reminding providers and patients when particular services are due. Finally, HIT makes it easier to record and analyze the performance of an intervention, so that the intervention can be improved over time. For example, one can use data collected on today's medical practices to develop still-better care guidelines.

The study has found, however, that there is not a straight line from installing information technology to reaping a benefit—not in healthcare (Scoville et al., 2005), and not in other sectors of the economy (Bower, 2005). Information technology is an *enabler*: It makes possible new ways of working and new processes (Hammer and Champy, 1993). But people do not inevitably adopt new ways of working just because they have a new information technology application. In this monograph, therefore, we have defined our interventions in terms of changes in the way the healthcare system behaves, and we have estimated the benefits of those changes in behavior. And as mentioned, we have discussed what roles HIT can play to facilitate these changes. But we know that implementing the "right" kind of HIT will not guarantee that the healthcare system will change in the ways we have postulated. Therefore, the reader should view our results as estimates of what *could* be, and not predictions of what *will* be.

Organization of This Monograph

We used a common set of large, publicly available healthcare data files to estimate effects of the interventions listed earlier. Our primary source was the Medical Expenditure Panel Survey (MEPS),[2] one of a series of national probability surveys conducted by the Agency for Healthcare Research and Quality (AHRQ) on the financing and utilization of medical care in the United States. Chapter Two describes how we created a database of patient trajectories from several years of the MEPS, a survey of the civilian, noninstitutionalized population by households. For each member in each household surveyed, it describes utilization, expenditures, and health status.

In Chapter Three, we compare the MEPS with other sources of data on utilization and expenditures. There are data sources that examine utilization alone, or expenditures alone, or population health status alone; the MEPS is the only publicly available source of data that puts them all together. However, the other data sources are often considered more accurate within their specialized domains. Thus, we devised adjustments to align our MEPS-based estimates with them. As well, we devised adjustments that project our estimates of the effects our interventions would have in the healthcare system of the year 2000 into the context of a future healthcare system. It is, however, a healthcare system that has only changed in ways foreshadowed by present trends. Chapter Three also explores how the healthcare system might change, if not by following present trends.

Next, we describe how we used information from the research literature to modify the trajectory database and produce estimates of the potential effects of the interventions listed above. Chapter Four discusses implementation of Computerized Physician Order Entry (CPOE) as a means of reducing adverse drug events in both hospital and ambulatory environments. In Chapter Five, we estimate the effects of influenza and pneumococcal vaccination, and of screening for breast cancer, cervical cancer, and colorectal cancer. Reminders provided by Electronic Health Record Systems have been shown to increase the likelihood that patients receive these services. Chapter Six estimates the costs and benefits of enrolling people with chronic illnesses in disease management programs. Effective disease management requires that the provider maintain a patient registry, and that enrolled patients have the means to receive advice and support from the provider, and to send current symptoms and questions to the provider, all in real-time. These functions are best performed by information technology.

Chapter Seven estimates the potential benefits of a program of lifestyle change in which everybody controlled their weight, stopped smoking, ate a healthy diet, exercised, and controlled their blood pressure and cholesterol as necessary with medications. In the long run, the population would be much healthier and it would use sub-

---

[2] Files and documentation for each year are available at http://www.meps.ahrq.gov.

stantially less healthcare. But for these outcomes to happen, consumers must come to see themselves as their own front-line caregivers. They need the information, the skills, and the confidence to keep themselves healthy to the degree they can, and to seek help when events slip out of their control. By itself, information technology will not bring about this transformation. But the transformation cannot happen without information technology.

Chapter Eight discusses what may be the most profound aspect of the HIT-mediated transformation of healthcare: requiring more of the patient or consumer (a person does not have to be sick to receive healthcare). Through disease management and lifestyle changes, healthcare ceases to be a commodity that healthcare providers deliver to passively accepting patients. Instead, it becomes an activity in which consumers and providers engage jointly and cooperatively.

In Chapters Four through Seven, we estimated potential benefits of our interventions. Chapter Nine compares the interventions in terms of their potential benefits, and the difficulty and likelihood of achieving the potential benefits in practice.

CHAPTER TWO

Building the Trajectory Database from the MEPS

James H. Bigelow, Ph.D., Kateryna Fonkych, and Constance Fung, M.D.

Introduction

A *patient trajectory* is the sequence of events that involves the patient with the healthcare system. For our analysis of the interventions listed in Chapter One, we have created a database of patient trajectories from several years of the Medical Expenditure Panel Survey (MEPS) (AHRQ, multiple years). The MEPS distinguishes the eight types of events listed in Table 2.1.

Our database also includes data from the MEPS files that describe the patient, such as age, sex, ethnicity, health insurance status, measures of health status, and medical conditions. Two of each year's MEPS files, the *Full Year Consolidated Data File* and the *Medical Conditions File,* are devoted to such information. Certain of the event files—prescribed medications, hospital inpatient stays, emergency room (ER) visits, outpatient department visits, and office-based medical provider visits—also include data on medical conditions.

Each year, the MEPS recruits a new panel of households. Households in a panel are interviewed five times over a 2.5-year period to collect two years of data on medical expenditures and utilization. Thus, in any year, households from two successive

Table 2.1
Types of Event Files in MEPS

Type	Title
A	Prescribed Medicines
B	Dental Visits
C	Other Medical Expenses
D	Hospital Inpatient Stays
E	Emergency Room Visits
F	Outpatient Department Visits
G	Office-Based Medical Provider Visits
H	Home Health

panels contribute data (Figure 2.1), and these data are combined to produce public-use files for that year. For example, extracts from panels 3 and 4 are combined to form the files for 1999.

For each panel *N*, there is a file (the *MEPS Panel N Longitudinal Weight File*) that contains a person-level weight for each respondent in the panel. These weights can be used to scale quantities recorded for individual respondents up to the level of the nation as a whole. For example, if respondent *j* has $ADMITS_j$ hospital admissions during the two years covered by the panel, then the total hospital admissions for the nation for those two years should be $\Sigma WT_j \times ADMITS_j$.[1]

To create the trajectory database, we combined data from panels 1 through 4 to obtain a set of analysis files with about 56,000 respondents. For most respondents, we had two years of data. The process has four parts, which we discuss in turn below:

- Develop person-level weights for each respondent, which let us calculate national-level quantities other than expenditures for our base year of 2000.

Figure 2.1
Overlapping-Panel Structure of MEPS

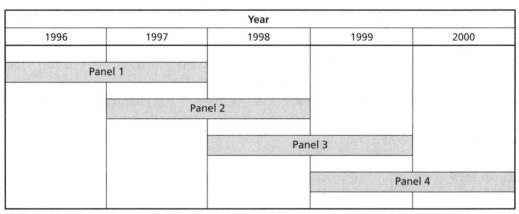

RAND *MG408-2.1*

---

[1] Originally, we anticipated that we would treat each two-year trajectory as a single observation, and this necessitated that each trajectory have a single weight, which we obtained from the longitudinal files. Ultimately, however, we treated each person-year of data as a separate observation, i.e., we broke each two-year trajectory into two observations, one for each year. Had we made this decision earlier, it would have been preferable to use the person-level weights provided in each *Full Year Consolidated Data File*, even though the same respondent would generally have a different weight in each of his/her two years. Data processing would have been simpler, and our analysis database would have had more observations (we would have kept the first year of data for panel 5 respondents, plus some respondents in earlier panels lost to follow-up in their second year) and slightly higher estimates of utilization and expenditures. Our results, however, would not have been markedly different.

- Inflate prices to the 2000 level so that we can calculate expenditures for our base year.
- Map the diagnoses in the MEPS into medical conditions that we have defined.
- Calculate health outcome variables.

Develop Person-Level Weights

In this section, we describe the sources and derivation of the person-level weights in our combined file. In brief, we adjusted the baseline weights in our combined file so that, when we summed the weights over all respondents, we obtained the total civilian, noninstitutionalized population for the year 2000 (which we have chosen as our base year). We calculated two multipliers that adjusted those weights to reflect the two major components of the institutionalized population: nursing home residents and inmates of correctional institutions. And we provided multipliers to inflate the 2000 population to 2005, 2010, 2015, and 2020.

Baseline Person-Level Weights

For each panel, there is a MEPS file of longitudinal person-level weights. We derived person-weights for respondents in our combined file from these longitudinal weights, as shown in Table 2.2. To adjust the weights to account for differences in the total populations, we multiplied a panel's weights by a population-growth factor, which is simply the ratio of the year 2000 population to that panel's population. To combine the four panels, we multiplied the weights for each panel by the fraction of total respondents that were in that panel. We combined the two factors into the single overall multiplier shown in the last row of the table.

We justify this procedure as follows. Estimating any quantity using these weights is equivalent to, first, estimating that quantity four times, once using the data for each panel. Each panel-specific estimate must first be adjusted for population growth, and then the four adjusted estimates must be combined into a final, overall estimate. To obtain a combined estimate with the minimum possible variance, the weights for the panel-specific estimates should be inversely proportional to the panel-specific variances. Since the MEPS design is similar from one panel to the next, one would expect panel-specific variances to be inversely proportional to sample size, and this is why we have multiplied the weights for each panel by the fraction of total respondents in that panel. Of course, each quantity one estimates will have its own panel-specific variances, and the variances will not all be inversely proportional to sample size. Overall, however, the rule should hold at least roughly. In any case, we know of no better rule.

Table 2.2
Source of Adjustment Factors for Longitudinal Person-Weights, by Panel

	MEPS File				
	Year 2000	Panel 1	Panel 2	Panel 3	Panel 4
Total Population (=sum of wts)	278,405,516	274,603,911	277,125,061	279,881,445	281,946,024
Population-Growth Factor		1.01384	1.00462	0.99473	0.98744
No. Respondents	25,096	19,859	12,445	10,122	13,316
Fraction of Respondents		0.35627	0.22326	0.18159	0.23889
Overall Multiplier		0.36120	0.22429	0.18063	0.23589

Adjustments to the Baseline Weights

For each respondent, we define seven multipliers that we can apply to the baseline weights to reflect various factors. Five multipliers inflate the 2000 population to future years: MULT00 (the multiplier equals 1), MULT05, MULT10, MULT15, and MULT20 inflate the population to the years 2000, 2005, 2010, 2015, and 2020, respectively. It is more convenient to include a multiplier for the year 2000 that is always equal to 1 than to treat that year as a special case.

The other two multipliers are MNURS, used to add nursing home residents, and MPRIS, used to add inmates in correctional institutions. Together, nursing home residents and inmates of correctional institutions accounted for over 90 percent of the institutionalized population in 2000 (3.7 million out of a total of just over 4 million).[2]

Adjusting the weights has the effect of increasing not only the population but also healthcare utilization and expenditures. The adjustment for nursing home residents ignores the cost of residing in the home, because these costs are deliberately not included in MEPS. It assumes that a nursing home resident will visit the hospital or a physician's office as often, on average, as a demographically similar person who is not in a home. One may question this assumption—after all, one reason people are in nursing homes is because they are too sick to stay home. But we have no data to support any other assumption.[3]

The adjustment for prisoners makes a similar assumption: that an inmate of a correctional institution will use the same amount of healthcare, on average, as a

---

[2] The Census Bureau classifies *institutions* as one kind of group quarters. Go to www.census.gov, click on "American Factfinder," then "Data Sets," then "Detailed Tables." As of December 19, 2004, the tool we found there asked us to select a geographical resolution and then a table, each from a drop-down list. The group-quarters tables are at the end of the list, labeled PCT17 and PCT17A-I.

[3] We felt it was important to account for nursing home residents, in particular, because they are such heavy users of healthcare. Unfortunately, our method for doing so undoubtedly underestimates their healthcare utilization, expenditures, disease burdens, and mortality. Further research to improve our estimates would be warranted. These adjustments add less than 3 percent to population, utilization, and expenditure totals. But they add 4 percent to the 75–84 age group, and 18 percent to the 85-and-over age group.

similar person who is not incarcerated. Again, we have no data to support an alternative assumption.[4]

We did not develop an adjustment for the active-duty military population (about 1.4 million people, as of 2000), because this population uses mostly facilities for their healthcare that are not used by civilians. Since we use the weights to inflate not only the population but also healthcare utilization and expenditures, we thought it best to omit the military population. (Veterans, of course, are civilians and are thus included in the MEPS, as long as they are not institutionalized.)

We did not create multipliers individually for each of the 56,000 MEPS respondents in our trajectory database. Instead, we defined 120 groups of respondents according to age, sex, and ethnicity, and developed multipliers for each group. Each respondent in a group was given the multipliers for that group. Table 2.3 shows the categories of age, sex, and ethnicity used to define the groups.

We formed the age categories from two different partitions of age. One was a standard set of 11 categories often used to report age-related data (e.g., mortality data and population projections). The 11 categories are as follows: less than 1, 1–4, 5–14, 15–24, 25–34, 35–44, 45–54, 55–64, 65–74, 75–84, and 85+. The other partition is one used by the Census Bureau to report the population living in group quarters. It uses three age categories: less than 18, 18–64, and 65+. The 12 age categories in Table 2.3 are constructed so that each one is entirely contained in one of the 11 and in one of the three categories of the other two age partitions.

Table 2.3
Population Groups Used for Adjustment of Person-Level Weights

2 Sexes	×	5 Ethnicities	×	12 Age Categories
Female Male		White, not Hispanic Black, not Hispanic Asian/Pacific Islander, not Hispanic American Indian/Aleut/Eskimo, not Hispanic Hispanic		<1 1–4 5–14 15–17 18–24 25–34 35–44 45–54 55–64 65–74 75–84 85+

---

[4] There is much less reason to adjust the MEPS data to include prisoners. Most of them are young and probably not particularly heavy users of healthcare.

Future-Years Adjustment

We aggregated Census Bureau projections of future-year populations[5] into 110 groups (2 sexes by 5 ethnicities by 11 age categories). For each future year of interest (2005, 2010, 2015, and 2020), we calculated the ratios of the population in each of the 110 groups to the number of people the Census Bureau estimated were in the group in 2000. To expand this set of 110 multipliers to the entire 120 groups defined in Table 2.3, we used the multipliers for age category 15–24 for both categories 15–17 and 18–24. To adjust the weight for a MEPS respondent so that it reflects a future year, we determined the group that contains the respondent and multiplied his weight by that group's ratio for the year in question.

Prison Population Adjustment

The tables for the group-quarters data from the Census Bureau that were our source for the prison population only give populations in three age groups (less than 18, 18–64, and 65+), so we used a partition of only 30 population groups (2 sexes by 5 ethnicities by 3 age categories). Each multiplier was the ratio of the appropriate population from the 2000 MEPS to the total population in that group in our combined file. To expand this set of 30 multipliers to the entire 120 groups defined in Table 2.3, we used the multipliers for prisoner age category "less than 18" for the first four age categories in Table 2.3; the multipliers for prisoner age category 18–64 for the next five age categories in Table 2.3; and the multipliers for prisoner age category 65+ for the last three age categories in Table 2.3.

Nursing Home Resident Adjustment

We obtained the 1999 nursing home population from the National Nursing Home Survey (NNHS).[6] We partitioned the nursing home population into 110 groups (2 sexes by 5 ethnicities by 11 age categories) and formed ratios of nursing home residents to baseline MEPS populations in each group. To expand this set of 110 multipliers to the entire 120 groups defined in Table 2.3, we used the multipliers for age category 15–24 for categories 15–17 and 18–24. We used these multipliers to inflate the MEPS person-level weights so that our estimates will include nursing home residents.

---

[5] Available from http://w w.census.gov/population/www/projections/natdet.html (downloaded January 4, 2004). There are low, middle, and high projections; we selected the middle one.

[6] Available from http://www.cdc.gov/nchs/about/major/nnhsd/nnhsd.htm (downloaded April 15, 2003).

Inflate Price

Each year of MEPS data yields different average expenditures per event for the various kinds of events that are listed in Table 2.1. We computed ratios of expenditures in 1996 through 1999 to the 2000 expenditures, and we multiplied expenditures on each individual event by the appropriate ratio (Table 2.4). Events that occurred in the same year to respondents from different panels were inflated by the same factors.[7]

Table 2.4
Inflation Factors by Expenditure Category

Expenditure Category	Year				
	1996	1997	1998	1999	2000
Office-Based Visits					
Total	1.278	1.279	1.208	1.146	1
Visits to Physicians	1.273	1.266	1.178	1.121	1
Visits to Non-Physicians	1.250	1.290	1.262	1.195	1
Hospital Outpatient Visits					
Total Facility Expense	1.120	1.033	1.002	1.041	1
Total Expense for Separate Providers	0.765	0.858	0.640	0.781	1
Facility Expense for Visits to Physicians	1.265	1.104	0.942	0.963	1
Separate Provider Expense for Visits to Physicians	0.952	1.004	0.661	0.745	1
Facility Expense for Visits to Nonphysicians	1.051	0.960	1.115	1.169	1
Separate Provider Expense for Visits to Non-physicians	0.596	0.655	0.607	0.875	1
Emergency Room Visits					
Total Facility Expense	1.152	1.052	1.174	1.108	1
Total Expense for Separate Providers	1.064	1.076	0.946	0.942	1
Hospital Inpatient Stays					
Total Facility Expense	0.943	0.997	0.978	0.978	1
Total Expense for Separate Providers	1.131	1.262	1.029	1.029	1
Dental Visits					
Total Expense	1.332	1.259	1.155	1.105	1
Home Health Care					
Agency Sponsored	0.976	1.007	1.096	0.803	1
Paid Independent	1.307	1.849	1.948	2.067	1
Other					
Vision Aids	1.163	1.373	1.234	1.131	1
Other Medical Supplies and Equipment	0.530	0.445	0.839	0.544	1
Prescription Drugs	1.329	1.226	1.186	1.030	1

[7] One would not expect these factors to agree with published inflation rates for individual components of healthcare, and we have not tried to compare them. Medical costs rise faster than prices because the technology, intensity, and other factors change as well.

Map MEPS Diagnoses into Medical Conditions

We defined 27 medical conditions, 20 of which we used in our subsequent analyses of the interventions listed in Chapter One (Table 2.5).[8] The definitions appear in the Chapters Four through Seven, in which we describe the analyses; we will not repeat them here. Here, however, we describe how we mapped the MEPS data into our medical-conditions definitions. The complete data can be found in the Microsoft Excel file MedicalConditions.xls at http://www.rand.org/publications/MG/ MG408/, and on the compact disc (CD) attached to the back cover of printed copies of this report.

The MEPS provides two codes for diagnoses. One consists of the first three digits of the 5-digit *International Classification of Diseases,* Revision 9 (ICD-9) code (we denote the three digits by ICD9.3). Because ICD-9 is a hierarchical code, the fourth and fifth digits do not entirely change the meaning of the 3-digit stub; rather, they add specificity. The other code, the Clinical Classification Code (CCC), was defined by the Agency for Healthcare Research Quality as an aggregation of 5-digit ICD-9 codes. If it were an aggregation of 3-digit codes, it would add nothing. Taking the ICD9.3 and the CCC together provides somewhat more specificity than

Table 2.5
Targeted Medical Conditions

Cancer of the breast
Cancer of the cervix
Cancer of the colon, rectum, and anus
Cancers of the head and neck, esophagus, and bronchus and lung (caused by smoking)

Cerebrovascular disease/Stroke
Congestive heart failure (CHF)
Coronary artery disease/acute myocardial infarction (AMI)
Hyperlipidemia
Hypertension
Other heart diseases

Asthma
Chronic bronchitis
Emphysema

Influenza
Pneumococcal diseases

Diabetes
Chronic renal failure (complication of diabetes)
Limb problems (complication of diabetes)
Retinopathy (complication of diabetes)
Neuropathy (complication of diabetes)

---

[8] Early in the project, we thought we could analyze the other seven conditions but ran out of time.

either code does alone. We have defined our medical conditions as aggregations of (CCC, ICD9.3) pairs.[9]

We matched the diagnosis codes in the annual MEPS *Medical Conditions Files* against our medical condition definitions to produce a 27-position array with a "1" in each position with a matching diagnosis. Nonmatching positions are set to "0." This array is specific to a particular respondent in a particular year, and we used it to identify people eligible for a disease management program or likely to be affected by a lifestyle change.

Certain MEPS event files—prescribed medications, hospital inpatient stays, ER visits, outpatient department visits, and office-based medical provider visits (see Table 2.1)—include diagnosis codes in their descriptions. For each of these event types, we also created a 27-position array with a "1" in each position with a matching diagnosis and zeroes elsewhere. These arrays were specific to a particular event (which, of course, occurred to a particular respondent in a particular year), and we used these arrays to identify the events (e.g., hospital stays, office visits, or prescription of drugs) most likely to be eliminated or changed by an intervention that targets that condition. For example, vaccinating people against influenza should reduce prescriptions for treating influenza.

Does this method select the right events or the right respondents? We conjectured that a respondent will have a medical condition (e.g., diabetes, CHF, influenza) if an event for that respondent mentions the condition. On the other hand, if a respondent has diabetes, for example, but never sees a doctor about it, he might not report it to the MEPS interviewer and we might not count him as a diabetic. Thus, we expected to undercount the number of people with each condition. We expected to undercount a lot for a condition such as influenza, for which most people do not seek medical care. We also expected to undercount mild cases more than severe cases of a condition—for example, mild asthma or CHF. In addition, we expected to undercount respondents with poorer access to health care—for example, the uninsured or underinsured.

A second source of error is the respondents. The MEPS is a survey of households, so it is a member of the household—a layperson—who reports the diagnoses associated with each event. It is not a provider, who we expect to have some expertise in making diagnoses. (A percentage of events reported by a respondent were cross-checked with the provider, which should mitigate the problem to some extent.) Edwards et al. (1994) compared household reports of chronic conditions with pro-

---

[9] We could define most of our conditions using the CCC alone. But in a few cases we split a CCC among several conditions. For example, we split CCC=127, "Chronic obstructive pulmonary disease and bronchiectasis" between Chronic Bronchitis (ICD9.3=491, "CHRONIC BRONCHITIS*") and Emphysema (ICD9.3=492, "EMPHYSEMA*"). Additional ICD9.3 codes were included in CCC=127 that we did not assign to any of our medical conditions. The asterisk (*) is included in the file of names for the ICD-9-CM (clinical modification) codes. Some conditions required several pairs for their definitions.

vider diagnoses and found that conditions that require a physician's diagnosis to identify show the highest agreement. These conditions include diabetes, most heart conditions, hypertension, and asthma. Once diagnosed, these conditions remain in the medical record and will continue to be reported on provider surveys. But they are likely to be underreported in a household survey. Edwards et al. suggest that heart disease is particularly subject to underreporting by households, because people with multiple conditions will lump them together.

Both Cox and Iachan (1987) and Johnson and Sanchez (1993) compared the diagnoses given for the same event by the household and by the provider. Both found that households give fewer diagnoses (in Johnson and Sanchez, only 10 percent of households associated more than one medical condition with an event, whereas 64 percent of providers did so). Both also found poor agreement between household diagnoses and provider diagnoses. As one would expect, if specific diagnoses were grouped into more general classes, the agreement improved.

We expect, therefore, that we have misclassified some respondents. That is, some respondents have a condition "in truth," but we say that they do not, and some respondents do not have the condition "in truth," but we say that they do. We make no general assessments of how large these errors may be. Rather, we address this issue for each condition at the point in the text where we first examine interventions that target that condition.

Calculate Health Outcome Variables

In subsequent chapters, we identify many Excel files containing extracts from the trajectory database. Each of these Excel files has a tab called "Outcomes." Here, we briefly describe the source of the outcome measures reported there.

All of the outcome measures are derived from data elements in each year's *Full Year Consolidated Data File*. We used the person status variables and the beginning and end dates of the interview rounds to set flags to indicate which respondents were "out of scope"[10] in parts of the two years, for each of several possible reasons: The respondent was born during the period, died, spent time in a healthcare institution or in a non–healthcare institution, spent time in the active military, spent time abroad, or some other reason. Of these reasons, we have reported only deaths in our Excel files.

Recall that information covering two years is collected from each household in a series of five interviews. The third interview covers parts of both years. We appor-

---

[10] A respondent can be included in the survey during part of the two years his or her panel is being interviewed, and excluded during other parts of the two years. When he or she is included, MEPS refers to him/her as "in scope." When he or she is excluded, he/she is "out of scope."

tioned missed days of work or school during this round in proportion to the number of days in the two years. We similarly apportioned days spent sick abed.

We calculated an activity-limitation variable from a number of the MEPS health status variables, using methodology described in Erickson, Wilson, and Shannon (1995). This variable takes on one of seven values: 1—Not limited in any way; 2—Not limited in major activities but limited in other activities; 3—Limited in a major activity; 4—Unable to perform a major activity; 5—Unable to perform instrumental activities of daily living (IADL) without help; 6—Unable to perform self-care activities of daily living (ADL) without help; and –1—Missing. It is defined differently, depending on the age of the respondent, and it may have a different value in each interview round.

We then calculated the fraction of each of the two years that the respondent had an activity limitation at each level. For convenience, we assumed that interviews 1 and 2 each covered 40 percent of year 1, and interview 3 covered the remaining 20 percent. Similarly, interview 3 covered 20 percent of year 2, and interviews 4 and 5 each covered 40 percent. If the five interviews reported activity limitations of (1, 1, 2, 2, 3), then we would say that for 80 percent of year 1 the respondent had an activity limitation score of 1, and for 20 percent of year 1 he/she had a score of 2. Similarly, in 60 percent of year 2, he/she had a score of 2, and in 40 percent of the year his score was 3.

In the same way, we calculated fractions of each year for which the respondent had each of the possible scores for perceived health status and perceived mental health status. These variables are provided in the MEPS Full Year Consolidated Data Files, and each of them has one of six values: 1—Excellent; 2—Very good; 3—Good; 4—Fair; 5—Poor; and –1—Missing.

CHAPTER THREE

Interpreting MEPS-Based Estimates

James H. Bigelow, Ph.D., and Kateryna Fonkych

Introduction

Those effects of interventions in the healthcare system that change patient trajectories, which we estimated in Chapter One, are changes in healthcare utilization (e.g., hospital stays, office visits, prescription drug use), changes in healthcare expenditures, and changes in population health outcomes (e.g., workdays or schooldays missed, days spent sick in bed). We have based our estimates largely on data from the Medical Expenditure Panel Survey (MEPS) (AHRQ MEPS, multiple years).

In this chapter, we discuss how these estimates ought to be interpreted. We considered four reasons for questioning what our estimates mean. The first is the precision of the estimates, as measured by standard errors. The second reason is errors and omissions, because the MEPS does not try to measure everything about the healthcare system. Parts of the system are left out—for example, long-term care. In the real world, the omitted parts would change, and we could not see these changes in our MEPS-based estimates.

Even the measurements it does make may contain systematic errors. For certain of our estimates, other sources of data are considered more accurate. For example, both the National Health Expenditures (NHE) and the MEPS provide estimates of healthcare expenditures, but the NHE is generally regarded as the authoritative source (Centers for Medicare and Medicaid Services [CMS] NHE). Thus, we have devised adjustments that align our estimates with more-authoritative sources of data.

Third, we estimated the effects our interventions would have in the healthcare system of the year 2000. In essence, we imagined that somebody changed the healthcare system back in, say, 1980, which would mean that the data collected by MEPS in 1996 through 2000 (the data we used to construct our trajectory database) would have been different. It is this difference that we attempt to estimate.

Contrast this estimate with what would happen in the real world. Our interventions would have to be implemented no earlier than the present, so in the real world we would see changes at least 15 years in the future, when we might reasonably hope to have changed the healthcare system. Thus, we have devised adjustments that project our estimates into the context of a future healthcare system. It is, however, a healthcare system that has only changed in ways foreshadowed by present trends.

Fourth, we speculated how the healthcare system might change if it did not follow present trends. Technological changes will flow from genomics, nanotechnology, and stem-cell research. Cultural attitudes may change, particularly about whether basic healthcare is a right and, possibly, about how much end-of-life care one is entitled to.

We also considered the well-known law of unintended (and unanticipated) consequences. A system is simply a collection of interacting parts, and, by means of those interactions, any initial disturbance will propagate throughout the system, often generating unforeseen effects. If the immediate effect of asthma management is to reduce hospitalizations, for example, hospitals may respond by trying to raise prices, reduce staffing, or drum up new business. We do not suggest that our estimates be adjusted for such effects. Rather, we suggest that these effects make our estimates uncertain, and we derive a range for that uncertainty. These effects take time to produce, so the uncertainty band is wider in years further in the future.

In the sections that follow, we discuss each of these four questions in turn.

Precision of Estimates from the MEPS Database

Tables 3.1 and 3.2 show the precision of selected utilization and expenditure measures estimated from the MEPS database. When estimates are made for the age categories shown, the relative standard errors of utilization measures (i.e., the ratios of the standard errors to the estimates) are smaller than 10 percent. The relative standard errors of expenditure estimates are somewhat larger, but still rarely exceed 15 percent.

We obtained our estimates of the standard errors in a manner that took into account the complex sample design of the MEPS. We used data from the MEPS 1996–2001 pooled estimation file[1] to assign respondents to strata and primary sampling units. These served as inputs to the Statistical Analysis System (SAS) SURVEYMEANS procedure, which uses the Taylor expansion method to estimate sampling errors.[2]

---

[1] Available at http://www.meps.ahrq.gov.

[2] Documentation for the SURVEYMEANS procedure is available online at http://v9doc.sas.com/sasdoc (last accessed April 27, 2005).

Table 3.1
Selected Utilization Measures and Their Precision

Age Category	Hospital Discharges		ER + Outpatient Visits		Office Visits to Medical Doctors (MDs)	
	Number (millions)	Relative SE	Number (millions)	Relative SE	Number (millions)	Relative SE
<1	0.61	8.8%	0.81	9.5%	12.90	5.3%
1–4	0.72	9.7%	5.16	5.2%	50.58	4.7%
5–14	0.86	9.6%	7.41	5.1%	71.79	4.2%
15–24	2.50	7.3%	9.80	5.1%	68.31	3.8%
25–34	3.28	5.9%	10.39	5.6%	97.12	4.4%
35–44	3.44	6.1%	13.74	5.0%	127.05	4.2%
45–54	2.89	5.4%	14.12	6.9%	125.15	4.0%
55–64	3.48	6.2%	10.94	6.6%	106.68	4.0%
65–74	4.28	5.6%	10.79	8.1%	115.40	4.4%
75–84	4.33	6.1%	8.28	6.4%	90.82	5.7%
85+	1.84	8.2%	2.26	8.6%	24.37	6.7%
Total	28.23		93.69		890.17	

NOTE: SE = standard error.

Table 3.2
Selected Expenditure Measures and Their Precision

Age Category	Expenditures on Hospitals		Expenditures on Physicians		Total Expenditures	
	Number ($billions)	Relative SE	Number ($billions)	Relative SE	Number ($billions)	Relative SE
<1	$5.19	16.5%	$1.63	8.2%	$7.09	13.6%
1–4	$4.68	13.0%	$4.84	6.4%	$12.46	8.0%
5–14	$6.45	9.5%	$7.86	7.7%	$32.27	6.0%
15–24	$17.22	15.4%	$11.50	5.7%	$44.55	8.0%
25–34	$19.23	9.4%	$16.14	5.0%	$56.12	5.9%
35–44	$27.23	6.5%	$21.58	4.2%	$81.64	4.4%
45–54	$28.77	6.7%	$21.09	4.6%	$87.47	4.5%
55–64	$39.66	9.4%	$20.24	4.7%	$91.27	5.8%
65–74	$40.00	5.8%	$20.20	4.7%	$91.80	4.4%
75–84	$46.66	9.7%	$17.39	7.0%	$92.99	7.1%
85+	$16.15	10.0%	$5.16	6.9%	$36.31	7.6%
Total	$251.24		$147.62		$633.97	

NOTE: SE = standard error.

Errors and Omissions in MEPS-Based Estimates

In this section, we discuss both the discrepancies between the MEPS and other data sources and the parts of the healthcare system that the MEPS omits but that other data sources include. Our estimates fall into three categories: utilization, expenditures, and outcomes. We discuss each in turn. Then, we discuss how to interpret our MEPS-based estimates in light of what we have learned.

Utilization Measures

The MEPS utilization data are specific. Each event—each hospital stay, each office visit—is described in considerable detail. The MEPS attaches each event to a person, so utilization can be related to any characteristic of the person who is included in the MEPS files: age, sex, ethnicity, medical conditions, health insurance status, employment status, income, and many others. For most types of events, the MEPS also attaches one or more diagnoses. Thus, we know the reason for each hospital stay and each office visit.

But are the MEPS utilization data accurate? The MEPS is a survey of consumers, and it is generally agreed that utilization data reported by providers is more accurate. Both the National Ambulatory Medical Care Survey (NAMCS) and the National Hospital Ambulatory Medical Care Survey (NHAMCS) are conducted annually by the National Center for Health Statistics (NCHS NAMCS; NCHS NHAMCS). The NHAMCS surveys hospital outpatient departments and emergency departments; the NAMCS surveys physician office- or clinic-based practices (thus excluding outpatient venues where one would not expect a physician to be present). Both surveys collect information on individual visits; there is no way to determine whether two or more visits were by the same patient. The Healthcare Cost and Utilization Project (HCUP) collects discharge summaries from hospitals and makes them available annually in the Nationwide Inpatient Sample (NIS) (AHRQ NIS). All the survey files include weighting factors on each visit or discharge, which can be used to generate national estimates of the various reported quantities.

Hospital Stays. Machlin, Cohen, and Thorpe (2000) compared estimates of hospital utilization made from five federal data sources, including the NIS and the MEPS. Their comparison used 1996 data, but the results were much the same as ours (Table 3.3).

There are three major discrepancies. First, the extraordinary difference in people under age 1 is due to the fact that the NIS counts discharges of healthy newborns as well as of their mothers, whereas the MEPS counts them as part of the

Table 3.3
Comparison of NIS and MEPS Hospital Inpatient Utilization

Age Category	NIS Discharges (millions)	MEPS Inpatient Stays (millions)	Error (MEPS – NIS)	Percentage Error
<1	4.69	0.61	–4.09	–87%
1–4	0.50	0.72	0.22	–44%
5–14	0.68	0.86	0.18	–27%
15–24	2.77	2.50	–0.27	–10%
25–34	4.01	3.28	–0.72	–18%
35-44	3.65	3.44	–0.21	–6%
45–54	3.68	2.89	–0.78	–21%
55–64	3.71	3.48	–0.24	–6%
65–74	4.92	4.28	–0.65	–13%
75–84	5.22	4.33	–0.88	–17%
85+	2.59	1.84	–0.75	–29%
Total	36.42	28.23	–8.19	–22%

same hospital stay. There were about 4 million births in 2000 (NCHS, 2003), and if these are subtracted from the NIS data or added to the MEPS data, the discrepancy for ages less than 1 disappears.

Second, even adjusting for this factor, the MEPS shows fewer hospital stays. Machlin, Cohen, and Thorpe (2000) think that the MEPS and other consumer surveys may systematically underreport hospital utilization. These surveys rely on recall by respondents over the previous several months, and respondents may overlook some hospitalizations. One might think that a stay in a hospital would be difficult to forget. But your hospitalization may not be too difficult for somebody else to forget, and MEPS interviewers frequently collect data for everybody in a household by interviewing just one member. Machlin and colleagues cite comparisons between the Medicare Current Beneficiary Survey (MCBS) and Medicare claims data that demonstrate underreporting in the Medicare population at least.

Third, the MEPS underestimate of hospitalizations is particularly pronounced among people 65 and older, which Machlin, Cohen, and Thorpe attribute to the fact that nursing home residents are excluded from the MEPS, and they are heavy users of healthcare. The MEPS estimates in Table 3.3 have been adjusted for the nursing home population, as described in Chapter Two. However, this adjustment assumes that nursing home residents are hospitalized at the same rate as people of the same sex, age, and ethnicity in the general population, which is an underestimate.

Emergency Room Visits. Machlin et al. (2001) also compared data on ambulatory visits from different sources. They found, just as we did, that the NHAMCS estimate of emergency room visits is twice as high as the MEPS estimate (Table 3.4).

Table 3.4
Comparison of NHAMCS and MEPS Emergency Room Visits

Age Category	NHAMCS (millions)	MEPS (millions)	Error (MEPS − NHAMCS)	Percentage Error
<1	4.06	0.49	−3.58	−88%
1–4	8.39	3.76	−4.63	−55%
5–14	10.94	4.94	−6.00	−55%
15–24	17.66	7.07	−10.59	−60%
25–34	16.70	6.54	−10.16	−61%
35–44	15.70	6.67	−9.03	−58%
45–54	11.20	5.08	−6.12	−55%
55–64	7.14	3.45	−3.68	−52%
65–74	6.54	3.18	−3.36	−51%
75–84	6.47	3.26	−3.21	−50%
85+	3.22	1.36	−1.86	−58%
Total	108.02	45.80	−62.22	−58%

Even when emergency room visits that result in a hospital admission are excluded, the NHAMCS figure remains twice as high as that of MEPS. Machlin and colleagues point out that the NHAMCS will capture visits by people that are not included in the MEPS, such as the homeless, residents of nursing homes, prisoners, and so forth (the MEPS estimates have been adjusted for prisoners and nursing home residents). Moreover, people who use the emergency room as their usual source of care may misclassify their visits to the ER as visits to the outpatient department or to a doctor's office or clinic. And MEPS respondents may simply not recall some visits, just as we suggested they may not recall some hospital stays. But it seems to us, as it does to Machlin et al., that the discrepancy is too large for these ad hoc explanations to be convincing.

Visits to Hospital Outpatient Departments. Machlin et al. (2001) found that the 1996 MEPS estimate of all visits to hospital outpatient departments was twice as high as the 1996 NHAMCS estimate. But many outpatient visits to hospitals are deliberately excluded from the NHAMCS. From the documentation provided with the NHAMCS, we learned that

> [outpatient] clinics were in scope if ambulatory medical care was provided under the supervision of a physician and under the auspices of the hospital. . . . Clinics where only ancillary services were provided or other settings in which physician services were not typically provided were out of scope.

Thus, a MEPS respondent who was sent to the hospital radiology department for magnetic resonance imaging (MRI) would report an outpatient visit to the MEPS interviewer, but such a visit would not appear in the NHAMCS.

A more appropriate comparison is between outpatient visits to physicians in the NHAMCS versus the MEPS. Machlin and colleagues found very good agreement when they made this comparison between the 1996 versions of the NHAMCS and the MEPS. When we compared our trajectory file with the 2000 NHAMCS, we did not get quite as good agreement (Table 3.5).

If we take the NHAMCS figures as "truth," then the MEPS underreports outpatient visits by young people and overreports visits by older people. We have factored in visits by nursing home residents at the same rate as people who are not nursing home residents, but it is plausible that nursing home residents would make more visits per person. Adjusting for this factor would merely accentuate the discrepancy at the higher ages.

Visits to Office-Based Providers. Machlin et al. (2001) found that the 1996 MEPS estimate of all visits to office-based providers was almost twice as high as the 1996 NAMCS estimate. But, once again, many kinds of providers are excluded from the NAMCS. From the documentation provided with the NAMCS, we learned that

> Only visits to the offices of nonfederally employed physicians classified by the American Medical Association (AMA) or the American Osteopathic Association (AOA) as "office-based, patient care" were included in the 2000 NAMCS. Physicians in the specialties of anesthesiology, pathology, and radiology were excluded from the physician universe.

By contrast, the MEPS specifically asks respondents about visits to nonphysician providers, such as chiropractors, nurses, or physical therapists. Such visits would be included in the NAMCS only if they occurred at the office of a physician in solo practice.

Table 3.5
Comparison of NHAMCS and MEPS Outpatient Department Visits to Physicians

Age Category	NHAMCS (millions)	MEPS (millions)	Error (MEPS – NHAMCS)	Percentage Error
<1	3.04	0.32	–2.72	–90%
1–4	4.98	1.40	–3.58	–72%
5–14	6.89	2.47	–4.42	–64%
15–24	6.63	2.73	–3.90	–59%
25–34	7.29	3.85	–3.43	–47%
35–44	8.59	7.07	–1.52	–18%
45–54	9.14	9.04	–0.10	–1%
55–64	7.39	7.49	0.10	1%
65–74	6.03	7.60	1.57	26%
75–84	4.17	5.02	0.85	20%
85+	1.27	0.90	–0.36	–29%
Total	65.42	47.89	–17.53	–27%

Thus, a more appropriate comparison is between office visits to physicians in the NAMCS and such visits in the MEPS. Machlin et al. found fairly good agreement when they made this comparison between the 1996 versions of the NAMCS and the MEPS. When we compared our trajectory file with the 2000 NAMCS, we obtained Table 3.6.

Except for infants (age less than 1), the results are quite consistent across age groups, although the excess visits in MEPS may be slightly more pronounced in the older age categories. The overall excess of 13 percent is slightly too large to dismiss as random error. The relative standard errors for both surveys are around 5 percent (see Table 3.1), so a difference of about 7 percent ($\sqrt{2} \times 5\%$) could be dismissed as random error. The actual difference is twice this large; nonetheless, we are going to ignore it. Although significant in a statistical sense, it is not important for our purposes.

Expenditures

The National Health Expenditures is generally regarded as the authoritative source for total healthcare expenditures. When a newspaper reports, for example, that national health expenditures in 2002 exceeded $1.5 trillion, the NHE is where they got the number. The NHE also provides the "official" definition of what is considered part of the healthcare system (CMS, 2001).

In this section, we compare the NHE with expenditures from the MEPS. We make the comparison for the 1997 files, because 1997 is the latest year for which the

Table 3.6
Comparison of NAMCS and MEPS Office-Based Visits to Physicians

Age Category	NAMCS (millions)	MEPS (millions)	Error (MEPS – NAMCS)	Percentage Error
<1	27.62	12.90	–14.72	–53%
1–4	44.27	50.58	6.31	14%
5–14	63.87	71.79	7.93	12%
15–24	63.49	68.31	4.82	8%
25–34	83.61	97.12	13.51	16%
35–44	104.90	127.05	22.16	21%
45–54	114.65	125.15	10.49	9%
55–64	93.56	106.68	13.12	14%
65–74	98.05	115.40	17.36	18%
75–84	74.82	90.82	16.00	21%
85+	18.76	24.37	5.61	30%
Total	787.59	890.17	102.58	13%

Bureau of the Census has published an economic census,[3] and we will be using the economic census data as a bridge between the NHE and the MEPS.

Table 3.7 shows total MEPS expenditures in 1997, in categories that the MEPS uses. The rows correspond to the types of events reported in the MEPS. The columns provide a breakout that will prove useful in the comparison below. Table 3.8 shows National Health Expenditures by type of expenditure for 1997.

Seven expenditure categories are included in the NHE but not in the MEPS. In 1997, these expenditures totaled $274.2 billion, or 25 percent of the overall NHE total. The remaining seven NHE categories of expenditures in Table 3.7 are included in the MEPS. The total of these categories in the NHE is $818.5 billion, compared with a total of only $563.6 billion for all 1997 MEPS expenditures.[4] In this section, we align the categories for the two sources—note that the MEPS records expenditures in different categories—and then compare them to see where the discrepancies arise.

Hospital Care. The NHE provides the official total national expenditures on healthcare, by line of Table 3.8. The MEPS includes only expenditures that reimburse directly for goods and services utilized by consumers. To determine how much of each line is related to utilization, we need more information. We turn to the economic census published by the U.S. Census Bureau. Data for the *1997 Economic Census* are the latest available.

Table 3.7
1997 MEPS Expenditures by MEPS Category

Event Type	Receipts by Recipient ($billions)				
	Facility	Physician	Non-MD Provider	Other	Total
Prescription medicines				$73.7	$73.7
Dental visits			$44.9		$44.9
Other medical expenses				$16.9	$16.9
Hospital inpatient stays	$192.2	$26.9			$219.1
ER visits	$14.6	$3.4	$0.1		$18.1
Outpatient department visits	$44.1	$8.4	$4.4		$56.9
Office-based medical provider visits		$81.5	$23.3		$104.8
Home health				$29.2	$29.2
Total	$250.9	$120.2	$72.7	$119.8	$563.6

---

[3] Data from the *1997 Economic Census* are available from the U.S. Census Bureau, http://www.census.gov/epcd/www/econ97.html. An economic census is performed every five years, and results for 2002 should be available shortly.

[4] Selden et al. (2001) noted that the MEPS total is much smaller than the NHE total (only 52 percent in 1997). They concluded that most of the difference arose from differences in which expenditures were included rather than from differences in estimates of comparably defined expenditures.

Table 3.8
National Health Expenditures in 1997 ($billions)

Type of Expenditure	NHE
National Health Expenditures	$1,092.8
Health Services and Supplies	1,055.5
Personal Health Care	959.2
Hospital Care	367.6
Professional Services	352.2
Physician and Clinical Services	241.0
Other Professional Services	33.4
Dental Services	50.2
Other Personal Health Care[a]	27.7
Nursing Home and Home Health	119.6
Home Health Care	34.5
Nursing Home Care[a]	85.1
Retail Outlet Sales of Medical Products	119.8
Prescription Drugs	75.7
Other Medical Products	44.0
Durable Medical Equipment	16.2
Other Non-Durable Medical Products[a]	27.9
Administration and Net Cost of Private Health Insurance[a]	60.9
Government Public Health Activities[a]	35.4
Investment	37.2
Research[a]	18.7
Construction[a]	18.5

[a] Category not included in MEPS.

The NHE hospital care category includes all enterprises with North American Industrial Classification System (NAICS) 3-digit code 622, Hospitals. The *1997 Economic Census* includes data on five kinds of enterprises with 3-digit NAICS code 622, as shown in Table 3.9. The two categories of government hospitals are tax-exempt, but the other three categories include both taxable (for-profit) and tax-exempt (not-for-profit) hospitals. There were a total of 6,685 hospitals of all kinds, with total revenues of $379.2 billion.

Table 3.9
Categories of Hospitals in the *1997 Economic Census*

NAICS	NAICS Title	Number	Revenues ($billions)	In MEPS?
6221101	General medical & surgical hospitals, government	1,591	$77.0	Yes
6221102	General medical & surgical hospitals (except government)	3,896	277.1	Yes
6222101	Psychiatric & substance abuse hospitals, government	262	8.8	No
6222102	Psychiatric & substance abuse hospitals (except government)	539	5.2	No
622310	Specialty (except psychiatric & substance abuse) hospitals	397	11.0	No

According to Selden et al. (2001):

The [NHE] contains expenditure amounts from non-community, non-Federal hospitals, which are out of scope [i.e., not included in] MEPS. Examples of such hospitals include mental hospitals providing long-term care of the sort not targeted by MEPS.

Thus, we estimate that only the general medical and surgical hospitals (the first two lines) are counted in the MEPS. The others are long-stay hospitals, and the MEPS should disregard most stays in them.

Table 3.10 shows the sources of the revenues of all hospitals. All of these sources except, we think, RL5300, Contract research, are included in the NHE category "Hospital Care." Thus, the total hospital revenues from the *1997 Economic Census* ($378.8 billion after excluding contract research) compare well with the NHE Hospital Care total ($367.6 billion—only 3 percent lower).

In the table, we allocate these revenues among three MEPS expenditure categories, plus revenues that are not in the MEPS. The columns for the three MEPS categories contain only revenues of general medical and surgical hospitals, which are the only ones that contribute to the MEPS. Further, only revenues for inpatient and outpatient services are counted in the MEPS.

Hospital revenues in the MEPS fall into three categories. They are facility expenditures for inpatient stays ($192.2 billion in 1997), ER visits ($14.6 billion), and hospital outpatient visits ($44.1 billion).[5] (In the table, the latter two categories are combined, because the *Economic Census* provides no means for separating them.) Inpatient revenues match almost perfectly. However, hospital outpatient revenues in the MEPS (the sum of ER and outpatient visits) are only 61 percent of the corresponding figure in the *Economic Census*. As we saw earlier, the MEPS greatly underestimates the number of ER visits and somewhat underestimates outpatient visits to physicians.

Revenues from home health care services are counted as hospital revenues in the *Economic Census* if the home health agency is owned by a hospital. In the MEPS, however, these revenues are dealt with as home health expenditures. We will encounter them below, when we discuss that MEPS category.

Physician and Clinical Services, and Other Professional Services. We treat these two NHE categories together, because neither one by itself maps conveniently to MEPS expenditure categories. The relevant MEPS categories are "physician revenues" and "revenues of non-physician providers." The NHE category "other

---

[5] These expenditures from the MEPS have been adjusted for the institutionalized population, as described in Chapter Two. The unadjusted numbers are $187 billion for inpatient stays, $14.3 billion for ER visits, and $43.4 billion for outpatient visits.

Table 3.10
1997 Hospital Revenues ($billions) by Source Code (*1997 Economic Census*)

Source Code	Kind of Business and Sources of Receipts	Inpatient Care	ER or Outpatient	Home Health	Not in MEPS
		MEPS Category			
RL5100	Payments for inpatient nursing and residential services				3.3
RL5150	Home health care services			4.8	
RL5200	Hospital inpatient services, except nursing home services	206.7			12.9
RL5250	Hospital outpatient services, except home health services		96.3		2.7
RL5300	Contract research				0.4
RL8500	Food and beverage sales (including cafeteria)				1.4
RL8550	Rental and leasing of goods and equipment				0.4
RL8600	Merchandise sales				0.4
RL8940	All other receipts				6.3
RL9000	Contributions, gifts, and grants. government				2.6
RL9050	Contributions, gifts, and grants (including individuals, community efforts, and commissioned fundraisers). Private				1.2
RL9100	Investment income, including interest and dividends				7.2
RL9150	Rents and commissions from departments and concessions not owned and operated by this institution				0.3
RL9200	Appropriations from general government revenues and intergovernmental transfers				26.9
RL9500	All other revenue				5.3
RL Total		206.7	96.3	4.8	71.3

NOTE: RL = revenue line.

professional services" contributes to nonphysician providers only; the "physician and clinical services" category contributes to both.

The NHE category "physician and clinical services" consists of NAICS 4-digit categories 6211, 6214, and part of 6215. The "other professional services" category includes NAICS 6213. These categories include the establishments in the *1997 Economic Census* that are listed in Table 3.11. The MEPS includes expenditures on all of these establishments. Table 3.11 lists the amounts these establishments contribute to the NHE.

The "physician and clinical services" category includes only the portion of medical and diagnostic laboratories' revenues that is billed directly to the patient. The remainder is billed to the medical provider, who will generally pass the cost

Table 3.11
Establishments in the *1997 Economic Census* That Contribute to Physician and Clinical Services (P&CS) and Other Professional Services

NAICS	NAICS Title	Number	Revenue ($billions) P&CS	Other Prof
621111	Offices of physicians (except mental health specialists)	219,069	$168.3	
621112	Offices of physicians, mental health specialists	11,103	$3.4	
621410	Family planning centers	5,010	$0.9	
621420	Outpatient mental health & substance abuse centers	11,943	$6.2	
621491	HMO medical centers	1,320	$14.0	
621492	Kidney dialysis centers	3,099	$4.9	
621493	Freestanding ambulatory surgical & emergency centers	3,152	$4.8	
621498	All other outpatient care centers	17,231	$18.0	
621511	Medical laboratories (part)	4,980	$7.0	
621512	Diagnostic imaging centers (part)	5,377	$3.9	
621310	Offices of chiropractors	44,364		$6.6
621320	Offices of optometrists	19,457		$3.4
621330	Offices of mental health practitioners (except physicians)	12,877		$2.5
6213401	Speech therapists & audiologists	3,697		$0.7
6213402	Physical & occupational therapists	13,842		$8.0
621391	Offices of podiatrists	11,955		$2.4
621399	Offices of all other miscellaneous health practitioners	7,263		$1.8
Total			$231.4	$25.3

NOTE: HMO = health maintenance organization.

along in his own bill to the patient. It would be double-counting to include this portion of laboratory receipts in the total healthcare revenues, since they are costs to one provider and revenues to another. From the 2001 Service Annual Survey,[6] we estimate that in 1997, a third of laboratory revenues are from healthcare providers and two-thirds are direct from patients. (By 2001, the percentage of revenues coming directly from patients had grown to about 72 percent.)

The *Economic Census* and NHE totals are very close for the "physician and clinical services" category ($231.4 billion versus $241.0 billion). For the "other professional services" category, the totals are closer in absolute terms, but with a larger relative difference ($25.3 billion versus $33.4 billion).

Table 3.12 again shows revenues for the NAICS codes in Table 3.11, but now allocated to MEPS expenditure categories. The "MD" column consists of patient care receipts paid to physicians; the "Non-MD" column contains patient care re-

---

[6] The Service Annual Survey is online at the U.S. Census Bureau, http://www.census.gov/svsd/www/sas62.html, sas62rpt.pdf, Table 8.15.

ceipts paid to nonphysician providers. The "Not in MEPS" column consists of revenues found in the *Economic Census* that are not patient care receipts. As noted earlier, the MEPS captures only expenditures that reimburse for services to patients.

Four MEPS expenditure categories correspond to the "MD" column of Table 3.12 and three to the "Non-MD" column, as shown in Table 3.13. The totals from MEPS are considerably lower than the totals from the *Economic Census.*

Table 3.12
Physician and Clinical Services and Other Professional Services Revenues ($billions) Allocated to MEPS Expenditure Categories

NAICS	NAICS Title	MD	Non-MD	Not in MEPS
621111	Offices of physicians (except mental health specialists)	$164.2		$3.9
621112	Offices of physicians, mental health specialists	$3.3		$0.1
621410	Family planning centers		$0.6	$0.4
621420	Outpatient mental health & substance abuse centers		$3.9	$2.4
621491	HMO medical centers	$12.5		$1.5
621492	Kidney dialysis centers		$3.9	$1.0
621493	Freestanding ambulatory surgical & emergency centers	$4.7		$0.1
621498	All other outpatient care centers		$14.1	$4.0
621511	Medical laboratories (2/3)		$6.9	$3.5
621512	Diagnostic imaging centers (2/3)		$3.9	$1.0
621310	Offices of chiropractors		$6.4	$0.2
621320	Offices of optometrists		$3.4	$0.0
621330	Offices of mental health practitioners (except physicians)		$2.5	$0.0
6213401	Speech therapists & audiologists		$0.5	$0.2
6213402	Physical & occupational therapists		$7.9	$0.1
621391	Offices of podiatrists		$2.3	$0.1
621399	Offices of all other miscellaneous health practitioners		$1.6	$0.1
Total		$184.8	$57.8	$19.5

NOTE: HMO = health maintenance organization.

Table 3.13
MEPS Expenditures ($billions) for Comparison with Physician and Clinical Services and Other Professional Services Revenues

MEPS Expenditure Category	MD	Non-MD
Separately billed hospital inpatient services	$26.9	
Separately billed ER services	$3.4	$0.1
Separately billed hospital outpatient services	$8.4	$4.4
Office-based services	$81.5	$23.3
Total	$120.2	$27.8

Dental Services. From Table 3.8, the NHE estimates an expenditure in 1997 of $50.2 billion on dental services, the NAICS 4-digit category 6212, which includes only a single kind of enterprise in the *1997 Economic Census*—621210, Offices of Dentists. The *Economic Census* lists total revenues for this enterprise of $48.5 billion in 1997. Virtually all of it was receipts for patient care. In the MEPS, expenditures on dentists were $44.9 billion in 1997. These three numbers agree very well.

We do not expect that our interventions would significantly affect expenditures on dental services. Thus, we do not consider these expenditures further in this monograph.

Other Personal Health Care. This category, which is not included in the MEPS, covers two types of expenditure: industrial in-plant services and government expenditures for medical care not specified by kind. *Industrial in-plant services* are facilities or supplies provided by employers for the health care needs of their employees. *Medical care not specified by kind* is delivered in nontraditional sites, such as community centers, senior citizens centers, schools, and military field stations. We do not expect that our interventions would affect these expenditures significantly.

Home Healthcare. From Table 3.8, the NHE estimates an expenditure of $34.5 billion on home health care in 1997. This category consists of the NAICS 4-digit category 6216, which includes only a single kind of enterprise in the *1997 Economic Census*—621610, Home healthcare services. In the *Economic Census,* there were 16,315 for-profit entities, which collected $21.5 billion in receipts, and 3,375 non-profit entities, which received $10.1 billion in revenues. The NHE category includes only freestanding home-healthcare enterprises. Hospitals collected $4.8 in 1997 for home healthcare services (see RL5150 in Table 3.10), which the NHE reports as part of the Hospital Care category.

The MEPS shows an expenditure of $29.2 billion on home health care. However, this includes home health care services delivered by hospitals, so it should properly be compared to the *Economic Census* number of $31.6 billion (for freestanding entities) plus $4.8 billion (for hospital-owned entities), or $36.4 billion. Once again, the MEPS estimate is substantially lower than either the NHE or *Economic Census* estimates.

Nursing Home Care. Expenditures reported as nursing home care are for services provided by freestanding nursing homes. These facilities are defined in the 1997 North American Industry Classification System as establishments primarily engaged in providing inpatient nursing and rehabilitative services and continuous personal care services to persons requiring nursing care (NAICS 6231) and continuing-care retirement communities with on-site nursing care facilities (NAICS 623311). The NHE includes hospital-based nursing home spending with Hospital Care expenditures.

MEPS does not include expenditures for nursing homes. MEPS covers only the civilian, noninstitutionalized population, and nursing homes are considered institutions.

Prescription Drugs. The NHE estimates an expenditure of $75.7 billion on prescription drugs in 1997. The total from the *1997 Economic Census* is $79.7 billion. The MEPS estimates $73.7 billion. All three estimates are identical, for practical purposes.

Durable Medical Equipment. *Durable medical equipment* includes contact lenses, eyeglasses, and other ophthalmic products, surgical and orthopedic products, equipment rental, and hearing aids. The NHE total for this category is $16.2 billion for 1997. The MEPS has a category called "other medical expenditures" that appears to contain expenditures for much the same kinds of items, and the total for this category was $16.9 billion for 1997. We found it impossible to separate durable from nondurable medical products in the *Economic Census,* so we do not present a number from that source.

Other Nondurable Medical Products. This category includes nonprescription drugs and analgesics, and medical sundries, such as rubber medical articles, heating pads, and bandages. It is not included in the MEPS.

Administration and the Net Cost of Private Health Insurance. This category has three parts. The net cost of private health insurance (the largest part) is the difference between the premiums earned by private health insurers and the benefits paid (which go into personal health care expenditures). The next-largest part comprises the administrative expenses of government programs, such as Medicare, Medicaid, and Workers' Compensation. Both federal government expenditures and state and local government expenditures are included. The smallest part comprises the administrative expenses associated with health activities of philanthropic organizations.

None of these expenditures is in the MEPS files.

Health information technology will have a substantial effect on these expenditures, as discussed in Girosi, Meili, and Scoville (2005). However, the Health Information Technology (HIT) applications they discuss do not change patient trajectories, and we do not consider them here.

Government Public Health Activity. Most federal public health activity emanates from the Department of Health and Human Services (DHHS). The Food and Drug Administration (FDA) and the Centers for Disease Control and Prevention (CDC) account for an overwhelming majority of federal spending in this area. State and local expenditures are principally those made by state and local health departments. Federal payments are deducted to avoid double-counting. Spending for environmental functions (air- and water-pollution abatement, sanitation and sewage treatment, water supplies, and so on) is excluded.

Public health expenditures are not in the MEPS files.

Health information technology could affect public health activities by making it easier to report and analyze cases of disease. However, these HIT applications were beyond the scope of our project.

Research. This category includes only research funded by non-profit or government entities. Research and development expenditures by drug manufacturers are not shown in this line, because those expenditures are treated as intermediate purchases under the definitions of national income accounting; that is, the value of that research is deemed to be recouped through product sales. The MEPS does not include research expenditures.

Health information technology could facilitate research by making it easier to collect and analyze data on treatments and outcomes. However, these HIT applications were beyond the scope of our project.

Construction. This category is limited to the value of new construction put in place for hospitals and nursing homes. It includes new buildings; additions, alterations, and major replacements; mechanical and electrical installations; and site preparation. Maintenance and repairs are excluded, as are nonstructural equipment, such as X-ray machines and beds.

Construction dollars are not in the MEPS files.

Outcomes

For most of the outcomes we estimated, there are no alternative sources of data available for comparison. Perceived health, perceived mental health, activity limitations, days of work or school missed, and days spent sick in bed are all available from the National Health Information Survey (NHIS), as well as from the MEPS. However, as with the MEPS, the NHIS is a population survey. (In fact, the households included in the MEPS are a subset of the NHIS households from the preceding year.) It does not offer a different perspective. Therefore, we have no reason to think that we need to adjust these outcome measures.

The Centers for Disease Control and Prevention collects mortality statistics with which we can compare deaths from the MEPS (see Table 3.14). It appears that the MEPS systematically underestimates deaths, but by only 14 percent.

We made the estimates in Table 3.14 using our MEPS data adjusted for prisoners and nursing home residents. Generally, prisoners are young; adjusting for them should not affect deaths very much. Adjusting for nursing home residents should have a larger effect, but our adjustment assumes that the death rate among nursing home residents is the same as that among people of the same sex, age, and ethnicity in the general population. This assumption surely underestimates deaths in nursing homes, and it could account for a substantial part of the shortfall, especially among people 85 and older.

Table 3.14
Comparison of Deaths in 2000 from CDC and MEPS

Age Category	CDC	MEPS	Error (MEPS − CDC)	Percentage Error
<1	28,035	6,975	−21,060	−75%
1–4	4,979	9,905	4,926	99%
5–14	7,413	3,358	−4,055	−55%
15–24	31,307	33,499	2,192	7%
25–34	40,451	18,794	−21,657	−54%
35–44	89,798	88,323	−1,475	−2%
45–54	160,341	123,176	−37,165	−23%
55–64	240,846	271,267	30,421	13%
65–74	441,209	377,378	−63,831	−14%
75–84	700,445	639,540	−60,905	−9%
85+	658,171	495,502	−162,669	−25%
Unspecified	356		−356	−100%
Total	2,403,351	2,067,717	−335,634	−14%

NOTE: Source of CDC deaths is (CDC, 2003b).

Adjusting MEPS-Based Estimates for Errors and Omissions

We have estimated the effects of interventions on healthcare utilization, healthcare expenditures, and population health outcomes. Here, we ask how to align our MEPS-based estimates with other surveys considered more reliable in their own domains—the NIS, NAMCS, and NHAMCS for utilization, and the NHE and *1997 Economic Census* for expenditures. (For economy, we will refer to these other surveys as "authoritative sources.") The adjustments are not intended to make total healthcare utilization, expenditures, and outcomes from the MEPS match the totals from these other sources of data. Rather, they are intended to make the changes in utilization, expenditures, and outcomes from the MEPS match the changes that we would hypothetically see in these other data sources in response to our interventions. Table 3.15 gives the alignment factors we have used.

Adjustments to Utilization Measures. Utilization estimates from the MEPS agree quite well with utilization from the NIS, NHAMCS, and NAMCS, except for hospital ambulatory visits. Inpatient stays and office visits to physicians need no adjustment. We combine ER and hospital outpatient visits, and multiply the MEPS estimates of their sum by a factor of 1.85, which is the ratio of NHAMCS to MEPS visit counts in Tables 3.4 and 3.5. We have no utilization estimates of visits to non-physician providers, except those from the MEPS; hence, we have no basis for adjusting them.

Adjustments to Expenditures. We adjust only hospital and physician expenditures. Table 3.7 gives hospital expenditures as $250.9 billion and physician expenditures as $120.2 billion in the 1997 MEPS. From the *1997 Economic Census,*

Table 3.15
Factors for Aligning MEPS-Based Estimates to
More-Authoritative Sources

Effect	Authoritative Source	Factor
Utilization Measures		
Inpatient stays	NIS	1
Inpatient nights		1
Hosp outpatient + ER visits	NHAMCS	1.85
Office Visits	NAMCS	1
Expenditures		
Hospital	NHE/ec97	1.21
Physician	NHE/ec97	1.54
Prescription drugs	NHE/ec97	1
Other		1
Days Affected		
Schooldays lost		1
Workdays lost		1
Total days abed		1
Mortality		
Deaths		1

corresponding expenditures on hospitals were $303 billion (Table 3.10) and corresponding expenditures on physicians were $184.8 billion (Table 3.12). The ratios of economic census numbers to MEPS numbers appear in Table 3.15.

Adjustments to Outcomes. We do not recommend making any adjustment to the MEPS-based outcome measurements. True, total deaths from the MEPS are 14 percent lower than deaths from the CDC data (Table 3.14). But there are large differences in deaths by age group. In the highest age groups, the differences are probably due to the nursing-home factor mentioned earlier. We do not know what factors may account for differences in lower age groups; indeed, the difference may be largely random rather than systematic.[7]

Projecting Estimates to Future Years

We have estimated the effects our interventions would have in the healthcare system of 2000, imagining that the interventions were introduced early enough that, by 2000, the healthcare system would have worked through any transients (i.e., effects of relatively short duration) and adjusted to the interventions. This conjecture is analytically convenient (which is why we do it), but it is not realistic. In this section,

---

[7] A total of 766 deaths occurred among the respondents in our MEPS database, but only 25 deaths in the ages 0–24 and only 39 in the ages 25–44. The Agency for Healthcare Research and Quality (AHRQ) advises that estimates should not be based on fewer than 100 observations.

we discuss the ways in which our estimates might be different if they were cast into the future, where they really belong.

Future Projections Based on Demographic Changes

Actually, we did take one step toward projecting our results into the future. As described in Chapter Two, we developed person-weights based on the Census Bureau projections, to reflect the growth and aging of the population. Table 3.16 shows the population in various future years, using those weights.[8]

From 2000 to 2020, the population grows by almost 16 percent, whereas the over-65 population grows by 52 percent, from 13 to 17 percent of the total. These demographic changes drive changes in utilization, expenditures, and outcomes.

Table 3.17 shows the effect of such growth on utilization. The effect of a population that is aging is plain. Even though the population as a whole grows by only 16 percent, hospital inpatient stays grow by 29 percent; outpatient department visits to physicians, by 28 percent; and office-based visits to physicians, by 21 percent. But the pattern of use remains as it was in 2000. There is, for example, no substitution of outpatient procedures for inpatient procedures, or of drugs for other forms of therapy.

Table 3.16
Population Projections (millions) for Future Years

Age Category	Future Year				
	2000	2005	2010	2015	2020
<1	3.8	3.9	4.1	4.3	4.4
1–4	16.2	16.3	17.0	17.8	18.4
5–14	40.4	40.4	40.2	41.2	42.8
15–24	38.7	41.3	42.7	42.2	41.7
25–34	39.7	39.0	40.9	43.2	44.6
35–44	45.2	42.8	39.4	38.7	40.5
45–54	35.5	39.5	41.1	38.7	35.5
55–64	23.3	28.6	33.8	37.6	39.3
65–74	19.0	19.7	22.7	27.7	32.4
75–84	13.4	13.9	13.8	14.4	16.9
85+	4.9	5.6	6.4	7.0	7.4
Unspecified	1.9	2.0	2.1	2.1	2.2
Total	282.1	293.3	304.2	315.1	326.1
65 and older					
Number	37.3	39.3	42.9	49.1	56.7
Percentage	13.2%	13.4%	14.1%	15.6%	17.4%

[8] All of our Excel files that contain results include data on projections of MEPS utilization, expenditures, and outcomes into future years. The tables in this section (Tables 3.14 through 3.17) were developed from I0D14mlt40.xls, which is available at http://www.rand.org/publications/MG/MG408, and on the compact disc (CD) attached to the back cover of printed copies of this monograph.

Table 3.17
Projections of MEPS Utilization for Future Years

Event Type	Future Year				
	2000	2005	2010	2015	2020
Inpatient Stays (millions)	28.2	29.8	31.7	33.9	36.3
ER Visits (millions)	45.8	47.6	49.3	51.1	53.0
Outpatient Department Visits to Physicians (millions)	47.9	51.7	55.2	58.5	61.4
Other Outpatient Department Visits (millions)	79.6	86.1	91.9	96.9	101.0
Office-Based Visits to Physicians (millions)	890.2	929.0	972.5	1,023.5	1,077.2
Other Office-Based Visits (millions)	365.1	376.9	387.6	399.1	411.8

Table 3.18 shows the effect on expenditures. Again, the effect of a population that is aging is clear. Even though the population grows by only 16 percent, expenditures on hospitals rise by 31 percent by 2020; expenditures on physicians, by 23 percent; and expenditures on drugs, by 27 percent. Total expenditures rise by 26 percent. Keep in mind, however, that these expenditures assume that both the utilization patterns (Table 3.17) and healthcare prices remain the same as in 2000. We know that they have not remained so in the recent past, and we do not expect them to remain so in the immediate future. But, if utilization patterns and prices remained constant, Table 3.18 shows the healthcare expenditures one should expect to see in future editions of the MEPS.

Finally, when we use the person-weights for future years to project outcome measures, we obtain Table 3.19. As before, the effect of an aging population is plain. Whereas schooldays lost grow by only 5 percent and workdays lost grow by 11 percent between 2000 and 2020, total days sick in bed grow by 22 percent and deaths, by 42 percent.

Table 3.18
Projections of MEPS Expenditures ($billions) for Future Years

Recipient	Future Year				
	2000	2005	2010	2015	2020
Hospital	$251.2	$268.7	$286.8	$306.9	$328.8
Physician	$147.6	$155.1	$163.0	$172.0	$181.3
Non-MD Providers	$33.0	$34.3	$35.6	$36.8	$38.0
Prescription Drugs	$94.1	$100.0	$106.3	$113.1	$119.9
Other	$108.0	$113.1	$117.9	$122.9	$129.0
Total	$634.0	$671.2	$709.5	$751.7	$797.0

Table 3.19
Projections of MEPS Outcome Measures for Future Years

	Future Year				
Outcome	2000	2005	2010	2015	2020
Schooldays Lost (millions)	175.6	178.8	180.0	181.6	184.3
Workdays Lost (millions)	623.4	647.9	668.1	681.0	691.1
Total Days Abed (millions)	1,332.2	1,406.5	1,476.0	1,546.5	1,625.5
Deaths (thousands)	2,067.7	2,255.4	2,449.7	2,670.5	2,935.0

The NHE Projections of Expenditure

The projections in Tables 3.16 through 3.19 are what we would expect the MEPS to look like in future years if the population grew and aged as projected by the Census Bureau, but if utilization patterns and price levels remained as they were in 2000.

We know of no official projections of utilization, but there are official projections of expenditure. To produce them, the Office of the Actuary (OACT) in the CMS combines projections for Medicare and Medicaid spending (based on actuarial techniques) with projections for private health spending based on a multi-equation structural econometric model.[9] Table 3.20 shows OACT's projected expenditures in categories that more or less align with those of Table 3.18, but including only the years 2000, 2005, and 2010 (the NHE projections are available only through 2013).

Table 3.20
Projections of NHE Expenditures ($billions) for Future Years

	Future Year		
Expenditure Category	2000	2005	2010
Hospital Care	$413.2	$585.8	$791.5
Physician and Clinical Services	$290.3	$412.0	$580.3
Other Professional Services	$38.8	$54.2	$76.3
Prescription Drugs	$121.5	$233.6	$396.7
Other MEPS[a]	$110.2	$147.1	$196.9
Total MEPS	$974.0	$1,432.7	$2,041.7
Total Personal Health Care	$1,135.3	$1,651.5	$2,360.7
Total National Health Expenditures	$1,309.4	$1,920.8	$2,751.0

[a]Includes the other NHE categories that are in the MEPS—dental services, home health, and durable medical equipment.

---

[9] The methodology is described at nhe-projections-methodology.pdf, online at http://www.cms.hhs.gov/ statistics/nhe (as of May 22, 2004).

Tables 3.21 and 3.22 show the percentage growth by expenditure component of our projections for MEPS data and of the NHE projections, respectively. When we compare them, we find that the NHE growth rates are much larger than ours.

Table 3.23 provides factors by which to multiply the projected MEPS expenditures in Table 3.18, to make them grow at the same rate as projected NHE expenditures. Doing so would make sense if the entire discrepancy in growth rates (i.e., the differences between Tables 3.21 and 3.22) were due to increases in the prices of medical goods and services, and none of it were due to changes in utilization patterns. They can be calculated directly from a comparison of 3.21 and 3.22 for the years up to 2010. For subsequent years, we used the NHE projections from 2010 through 2013 to develop annual growth rates for each expenditure component, assuming these rates would apply to all years after 2010.

These factors do not adjust for the differences between the MEPS and NHE estimates in the year 2000. Thus, they should be applied in addition to the alignment factors in Table 3.15.

Projecting Future Utilization

Heffler et al. (2004) have attributed the growth in projected NHE expenditures to four factors. Looking at their Exhibit 6, medical prices appear to grow at about 3.8 percent per year from 2004 to 2013. They split demographic effects into two parts, an effect due to the change on overall population size (a population effect), and an effect due to changes in the distribution over age and sex (an age-sex effect). The former drives expenditures up by 0.9 percent per year; the latter drives them up by only 0.3 percent per year. (By comparison, Table 3.18 shows that demographic changes increase expenditures by just over 1 percent per year, counting changes in both the size and age-sex-ethnicity distribution of the population.) Changes in utilization drive expenditures up by 2.2 percent per year, for a total growth of 7.2 percent per year.

Table 3.21
Cumulative MEPS Expenditure Growth

| Recipient | Future Year | | | | |
	2000	2005	2010	2015	2020
Hospital	0.0%	6.9%	14.1%	22.2%	30.9%
Physician	0.0%	5.1%	10.5%	16.5%	22.8%
Non-MD Providers	0.0%	4.0%	7.8%	11.6%	15.4%
Prescription Drugs	0.0%	6.2%	12.9%	20.1%	27.4%
Other	0.0%	4.7%	9.1%	13.8%	19.4%
Total	0.0%	5.9%	11.9%	18.6%	25.7%

Table 3.22
Cumulative Growth of NHE Expenditures in Future Years

	Future Year		
Expenditure Category	2000	2005	2010
Hospital Care	0.0%	41.8%	91.6%
Physician and Clinical Services	0.0%	41.9%	99.9%
Other Professional Services	0.0%	39.7%	96.6%
Prescription Drugs	0.0%	92.2%	226.4%
Other MEPS	0.0%	33.5%	78.6%
Total MEPS	0.0%	47.1%	109.6%
Total Personal Health Care	0.0%	45.5%	107.9%
Total National Health Expenditures	0.0%	46.7%	110.1%

Table 3.23
Escalation Factors That Make MEPS Projections Agree with NHE Projections

	Future Year				
Recipient	2000	2005	2010	2015	2020
Hospital	0.0%	32.6%	67.8%	106.7%	154.5%
Physician	0.0%	35.1%	81.0%	135.1%	205.4%
Non-MD Providers	0.0%	34.3%	82.3%	144.2%	227.4%
Prescription Drugs	0.0%	80.9%	189.1%	326.3%	530.8%
Other	0.0%	27.4%	63.7%	106.7%	159.6%
Total	0.0%	38.9%	87.3%	144.5%	218.9%

However, changes in utilization need not be simple growth in numbers of office visits or hospital stays. Utilization changes include changes in quality and mix of services. For example, every so often a new MRI machine is introduced with higher resolution than the older machines. Typically, the price of an image taken with the new machine will be higher than that of a lower-resolution image taken with last year's machine. That a different service has been rendered indicates, at least in part, a change in utilization, not just a rise in price.

Such utilization changes may not show up in the crude utilization measures we are using (see Table 3.17). In fact, in the decade from 1990 to 2000, per-capita office-based physician visits, per-capita emergency room visits, and per-capita hospital stays hardly changed at all (Bernstein et al., 2003). Per-capita visits to hospital outpatient departments increased by 29 percent from 1992–1993 through 2000.

Bernstein et al. (2003) do note changes in some characteristics of utilization. Office-based visits to physicians have gotten slightly longer (from 16.7 minutes in

1990–1991 to 18.1 minutes in 2000), and hospital stays have gotten shorter (from 6.4 days in 1990–1991 to 4.9 days in 2000). This trend toward shorter hospital stays has been accompanied by an increase in hospital transfers to nursing homes (from 4.3 percent of live discharges in 1985 to 8.5 percent in 2000).

Given this discussion, we see no reason to adjust our future-year estimates of effects on utilization or outcomes.

Factors Not Included in These Adjustments

Any future projection is a guess, and the projections on which we have based our adjustments of the preceding section are no exception. As with many projections, they are based on an analysis of recent trends. In this final section of the chapter, we discuss some factors that might upset those trends.

Technology

We now have a human genome database, courtesy of the Human Genome Project. That database is expected to lead to advances in molecular medicine, cures or therapies for many diseases, and drugs tailored to specific individuals.

Using nanotechnology, the country could potentially build machines the size of large molecules (and much smaller than cells) to do very specific tasks. The research team did a brief Google™ search and found the following potential tasks: (1) recognizing and killing cancer cells; (2) providing oxygen to regions with low blood flow (from molecular bottles containing oxygen at high pressure); and (3) acting as artificial mitochondria.

A short time ago, California voted to provide funding for stem-cell research. Proponents claim that such research will lead to cures for spinal-cord injuries, Parkinson's disease, Alzheimer's disease, and diabetes.

Might these factors utterly change the Health Information Technology (HIT) equation? One can speculate that, in a generation or less, the country will have individualized drugs and nanotechnological implants that will keep its citizens healthy in spite of unhealthy habits, such as eating junk food, smoking, and gaining weight. But such changes will probably not happen quickly, and many of them may not happen at all. Some pretty amazing things will probably happen, but chances are they will bring with them problems and disadvantages, as well as benefits. And there is no reason to think they will be "plug-and-play" inventions. It will take substantial skill and information to use them effectively. We are confident that they will require, if anything, an expanded role for HIT.

Cultural Attitudes

There is general agreement, at least in the press, that people are entitled to some basic level of healthcare. However, as shown by the existence of 45 million people with no health insurance, the country has not taken this attitude from wish to reality. Indeed, universal healthcare may not happen until the United States decides that it is acceptable to ration healthcare. At present, many believe that everybody is entitled to the best that medicine has to offer. You have to pay for a private room out of your own pocket, but you have a right—at least if covered by Medicare—to open-heart surgery at taxpayer expense. Ten or 15 years ago, the state of Oregon tried to construct a priority scheme for Medicaid recipients. They listed diagnoses and procedures in priority order, and proposed to pay for only the top part of the list, going down to the point where their budget ran out—causing a major outcry.

At present, people consume an enormous amount of healthcare at the end of life. Many people have asked whether this makes sense, and in other industrial countries they have mostly decided that it does not. In the Netherlands, assisted suicide is an option. From time to time, offering this option has been debated in the United States, although the debate seems rather muted just at present. But voices will rise again, and if Americans decide that basic healthcare is an entitlement, perhaps aggressive end-of-life care will not be considered part of the basic package.

Changes such as these would make a huge difference in healthcare. Extending healthcare to the uninsured might not cost an extraordinary amount of money—Hadley and Holahan (2003) estimate no more than $70 billion per year—but it would pose a challenge for continuity of care (the lives of the poor are often unstable). Changing attitudes toward end-of-life care could change total health care utilization and expenditures by enormous amounts.

Indirect Effects

A system, such as the healthcare system, is a collection of interacting parts. Any intervention that changes one part of the system will propagate by means of these interactions to other, perhaps remote, parts of the system. If the initial disturbance is small, its effects may not be noticeable very far (in space or time) from the initial disturbance. But if the initial disturbance is large, the effects may propagate far and persist for a long time.

The disturbance created by technology could be large. So, too, could the disturbance caused by changes in cultural attitudes. We judge some but not all of the interventions we consider to have the potential for large effects. Thus, widespread adoption of healthy lifestyle habits would be a very large disturbance. Universal adoption of disease management for chronic conditions would be large, as well. Reducing adverse drug events through Computerized Physician Order Entry (CPOE) adoption is, we think, a small disturbance. Increasing the provision of preventive services (e.g., influenza vaccination and *Papanicolaou* [PAP] smears) is also small.

The healthcare system can respond in different ways to these disturbances, and one can develop a sense of the range of possible responses by examining the variation in healthcare in different parts of the country. The *Dartmouth Atlas of Health Care 1999* (Wennberg and Cooper, eds., 1999) provides an in-depth look for Medicare enrollees. In 1996, total reimbursements per capita varied by a factor of 2.9 over the 306 hospital referral regions in the country.[10] Reimbursements for specific kinds of services (e.g., hospital care, professional and laboratory services) show similar variability. Adjusting for age, sex, race, illness, and prices has virtually no effect on the range of variation.

Rates of hospitalization of Medicare patients for medical (as opposed to surgical) conditions vary by a factor of 2.5 across hospital referral regions, from 134.3 hospitalizations per 1,000 enrollees in Salem, Oregon, to 330.3 hospitalizations per 1,000 enrollees in Meridian, Mississippi. Regional differences in the distributions of age, sex, race, and illness explain a variation of only about 1.5. The *Atlas* points out that for many conditions, medical science and theory are weak, and it is not clear what the best care is. Different physicians will prescribe different treatments, for reasons that seem good to them at the time.

The amount of healthcare provided in the last six months of life showed equally large variations. Table 3.24 shows the minimum and maximum values (taken over the 306 hospital referral regions) for selected indicators of the intensity of end-of-life care.

Table 3.24
Variation in Intensity of End-of-Life Care of Medicare Decedents in 1995–1996

Intensity Measure	Minimum	Maximum	Ratio
Percentage of Medicare Deaths Occurring in Hospitals	17.2%	49.0%	2.8
Percentage of Medicare Enrollees Admitted to Intensive Care During the Last Six Months of Life	14.2%	49.3%	3.5
Percentage of Medicare Enrollees Spending Seven or More Days in Intensive Care During the Last Six Months of Life	2.9%	25.5%	8.9
Percentage of Medicare Enrollees Admitted to Intensive Care During the Terminal Hospitalization	6.3%	29.0%	4.6
Physician Visits per Decedent During the Last Six Months of Life	8.5	47.9	5.6
Primary Care Physician Visits per Decedent During the Last Six Months of Life	4.5	19.0	4.2
Medical Specialist Visits per Decedent During the Last Six Months of Life	2.0	25.1	12.4
Percentage of Medicare Enrollees Seeing Ten or More Physicians During the Last Six Months of Life	1.3%	34.7%	26.4
Price-Adjusted Reimbursements for Inpatient Care During the Last Six Months of Life, per Decedent	$6,198	$17,797	2.9

---

[10] *Hospital referral regions* are the geographical units into which the *Dartmouth Atlas* aggregates its data. Maps of the regions appear in an appendix in Wennberg and Cooper, eds. (1999).

The *Atlas* finds some support for the theory that healthcare utilization is driven by supply rather than need. Thus, a region with a shortage of primary care physicians might see a higher-than-average rate of hospitalization of chronic obstructive pulmonary disease (COPD) and asthma patients. But the *Atlas* found that, while hospitalization rates for what they called "ambulatory care–sensitive conditions" varied by a factor of almost 3, the variations did not relate to access to or continuity of care, nor to the supply of primary care physicians. Rather, most of the variation was related to the supply of hospital beds.

The *Atlas* finds little support for the hypothesis that more health care equates to better health outcomes. Thus, if healthcare providers knew much more about which treatments worked for which patients, it is likely that they could squeeze most of this variation out of the system. The result would be a system that produced better outcomes at lower cost. But providers do not have this knowledge at present. Consequently, the system treats similar patients in a variety of ways, each way with its own defenders. It is not difficult to imagine that if there were a disturbance to the healthcare system in a region—say, a large reduction in demand for hospitalizations—then the system in that region could respond by adopting a different treatment pattern, one more like the pattern in another region.

Response 1: Blunt the Savings. To see possible indirect effects of a large disturbance, suppose that the number of cases that have historically resulted in a hospitalization drops by 30 percent over a 15- to 20-year period. One possible response is for hospital stays to drop by 30 percent and for 30 percent of hospitals (or hospitals totaling 30 percent of beds) to go out of business. But this possibility is not likely to appeal to hospital administrators, doctors, nurses, or anybody else whose livelihood depends in part on hospital revenues. Moreover, it is not the only possible response.

A hospital can try to persuade physicians that cases that heretofore did not call for hospitalization can be better treated in a hospital. The variation in hospitalization rates cited in the *Atlas* shows that this possibility is not far-fetched.

If the hospital can persuade payers that doing so is desirable, payers might increase the resources spent on each hospital stay. For example, in 1999, California passed a law that specified minimum ratios of nurses to patients in the various kinds of hospital units, ensuring that the number of nurses in hospitals decline by less than the hospital stays. (Needleman et al. [2001] provide some evidence that increasing nurses in hospitals improves patient outcomes.) As another example, hospital lengths of stay have been declining since the early 1980s; however, recently there has been something of a backlash (Bernstein et al., 2003). Hospitals might persuade payers to allow longer stays.

Physicians, too, have many opportunities to find new work to offset a loss of old business. Primary care physicians frequently complain that they cannot spend enough time with each patient. Indeed, this has been offered as one reason that physicians do not provide as much preventive care as the United States Preventive Services Task Force (USPSTF) recommends (Yarnell et al., 2003). A decrease in the number of office visits to physicians might simply result in more services performed per visit. Physicians can also call patients back for follow-up visits or refer patients to specialists.

Response 2: Embrace the Savings. The above examples show how the system could blunt the effects of changes to the healthcare system. But the opposite effect is also possible. The rapid rise in healthcare expenditures has provoked a proposal for health savings accounts. The idea behind them is to require the consumer to pay a significant fraction of his or her healthcare costs, up to some catastrophic limit. This, it is thought, will motivate the consumer to use only those healthcare services that will benefit him or her, thereby reducing overall utilization. Even without a financial incentive, there is some evidence that, when consulted, patients sometimes want less care than the doctor recommends. The *Atlas* reports such a phenomenon for discretionary transurethral prostatectomies (Wennberg and Cooper, 1999, p. 226). Concerning end-of-life care, the *Atlas* remarks that (pp. 232–234)

> [m]ost patients appear to prefer less intensive care at the end of life, and those who live in regions with lower intensity of care are more likely to receive the care they say they want (which is generally less than most people now receive). It is reasonable to use those regions in which the intensity of end of life care is low as "best practice" benchmarks of efficiency, because in those areas, lower spending results in no known loss of benefit, and appears to reflect patient preferences for end of life care.

Therefore, to the degree that the healthcare system adopts a more patient-centric paradigm, we may see an evolution toward less rather than more utilization of healthcare.

Finally, we ask how these considerations ought to affect our view of the estimates we make of the effects of interventions. In the *Atlas,* measures that apply to small populations can have startlingly large variations, but the more general measures typically vary by factors of 2 to 3—a reasonable range for our uncertainty. We think of these indirect effects as accruing over time, meaning that they will show up as increases or decreases in the growth rates of healthcare expenditures. We also think that they will apply to both the effects of interventions and to the baseline (i.e., what will happen in the absence of any interventions). The NHE projects a 6.7-percent growth rate from 2010 through 2013 for the expenditure components that are included in the MEPS. We calculate that the rate could be as low as 4.3 percent or as high as 9.2 percent, depending on whether the system responds to changes by embracing or blunting the potential savings. These two rates bracket the NHE rate, and 20 years of growth at 9.2 percent produces a result 2.5 times larger than the same 20 years of growth at 4.3 percent.

CHAPTER FOUR

Avoiding Adverse Drug Events Through Computerized Physician Order Entry

James H. Bigelow, Ph.D., and Constance Fung, M.D.

Introduction

Evidence suggests that Computerized Physician Order Entry (CPOE) can improve patient safety in both hospital and ambulatory environments (Bates, Leape et al., 1998; Bates, Teich et al., 1999; Johnston et al., 2003, 2004; Leape et al., 1995, 2000; Overhage, Tierney, and Zhou, 1997). Unsurprisingly, then, interest in CPOE increased greatly when the Institute of Medicine (IOM) (Corrigan and Donaldson, eds., 1999) reported that between 44,000 and 98,000 people die from medical errors in U.S. hospitals each year. The Leapfrog Group[1] has made installing CPOE in hospitals one of its recommendations (Birkmeyer et al., 2000, 2001).

One measure of patient safety is the incidence of adverse drug events (ADEs). These are injuries resulting in a medical intervention related to a drug (Bates et al., 1995). In this chapter, we describe how we estimated the effects of using CPOE in hospitals and physician practices nationwide to avoid both inpatient and ambulatory ADEs. In addition, we were able to estimate some benefits of ambulatory CPOE that are not related to ADE avoidance.

Computerized Physician Order Entry

When a hospital or a physician's practice implements CPOE, physicians stop writing orders by hand on pieces of paper and start entering them electronically into a computer system. But much more than order-writing is going on. First, the CPOE makes information available to the physician at the time he or she enters the order. If the

---

[1] The Leapfrog Group is

> an initiative driven by organizations that buy health care who are working to initiate breakthrough improvements in the safety, quality and affordability of healthcare for Americans. It is a voluntary program aimed at mobilizing employer purchasing power to alert America's health industry that big leaps in health care safety, quality and customer value will be recognized and rewarded.

Quote from http://www.leapfroggroup.org (as of February 17, 2005).

physician is writing a medication order, for example, the CPOE may present a list of drugs that the patient is already taking and warn of any interactions those drugs may have with the drug being ordered. The CPOE may display the patient's most recent laboratory results. It can check the dose against dosage standards. Once the order has been entered, the system can track the steps involved in executing the order,[2] providing a mechanism for identifying and eliminating errors. In the longer term, it provides the information needed to redesign the order-execution process so that making errors becomes much more difficult.

To provide these benefits, the CPOE must include decision support and it must have access to current patient-specific information—in effect, an Electronic Medical Record (EMR). Thus, when we speak of *CPOE,* we mean the capability of a more comprehensive health information system.

Implementing such a clinical information system is not merely an information technology (IT) project. It is an organizational-change initiative. As suggested by the comments above on order-execution tracking, the organization should anticipate that processes will have to change to take advantage of CPOE's potential. However, these changes can take place mostly within existing organizations. If a hospital installs CPOE, the value of CPOE can be realized by changing processes (such as the medication-administration process) within the hospital. It is not necessary that activities in the hospital be any better coordinated with activities at physicians' offices than they are now.

Adverse Drug Events

Bates et al. (1995) suggest what has become standard terminology for discussing adverse drug events:

- *Adverse drug events* are injuries resulting from medical interventions related to a drug.
- *Adverse drug reaction* is a synonym for adverse drug event.
- *Medication errors* are errors in the process of ordering or delivering a medication, regardless of whether an injury occurred or the potential for injury was present.
- *Potential ADEs* are medication errors judged to have the potential for injury but in which no injury occurred.
- *Serious medication errors* are medication errors associated with ADEs and potential ADEs.

---

[2] Currently, hospital CPOE systems are more likely than ambulatory systems to track execution, because executing in the hospital is the job of hospital staff. In the ambulatory setting, executing a medication order is the responsibility of the patient. Considering how many prescriptions go unfilled, and how many discrepancies there are between what the doctor prescribes and what the ambulatory patient actually does (Bedell et al., 2000), tracking would probably be a good idea in the ambulatory setting, as well.

Only a small fraction of medication errors is serious. Bates, Miller et al. (1999) report that in three medical units at Brigham and Women's Hospital, during four periods totaling 220 days in 1992–1997, a total of 2,363 medication errors occurred, of which 253 were deemed serious. Of the 253 serious medication errors, 216 were intercepted, meaning that they were corrected before the medication was administered to the patient. This left 37 nonintercepted serious medication errors, or about 1.5 percent of the total medication errors.

ADEs and medication errors are related, since some medication errors result in ADEs. But either can occur without the other. For example, if a patient has an allergic reaction to a drug and there is no record of his sensitivity, there has been an ADE but no error. Conversely, if a patient receives the wrong drug or the wrong dose but no injury results, there has been an error but no ADE. CPOE reduces ADEs by reducing medication errors. However, ADEs that are not the result of any error will occur despite the presence of CPOE.

The Inpatient Setting

We used the process shown in Figure 4.1 to estimate the effects of inpatient CPOE for the nation as a whole. Our data sources are listed across the top of the figure.

Opportunity and Frailty Scores

In our model, we assumed an overall rate for serious medication errors and for ADEs, and we needed to devise a way to distribute them among hospital inpatients having different characteristics. When Bates, Teich et al. (1999) attempted to identify patient risk factors for ADEs, he concluded that

> [a]dverse drug events occurred more frequently in sicker patients who stayed in the hospital longer. However, after controlling for level of care and pre-event length of stay, few risk factors emerged.

To capture the "sicker-patient" effect, we summarized the 1999 Medical Expenditure Panel Survey (MEPS) data to generate a list of patients grouped by diagnosis. A physician assigned opportunity and frailty scores based on these diagnoses. We intended the opportunity score for a diagnosis to reflect the relative likelihood that a hospital would make a serious medication error for a patient with that diagnosis. Each score could have values low, medium, or high.

Figure 4.1
Process for Estimating Effects of Using CPOE to Reduce ADEs

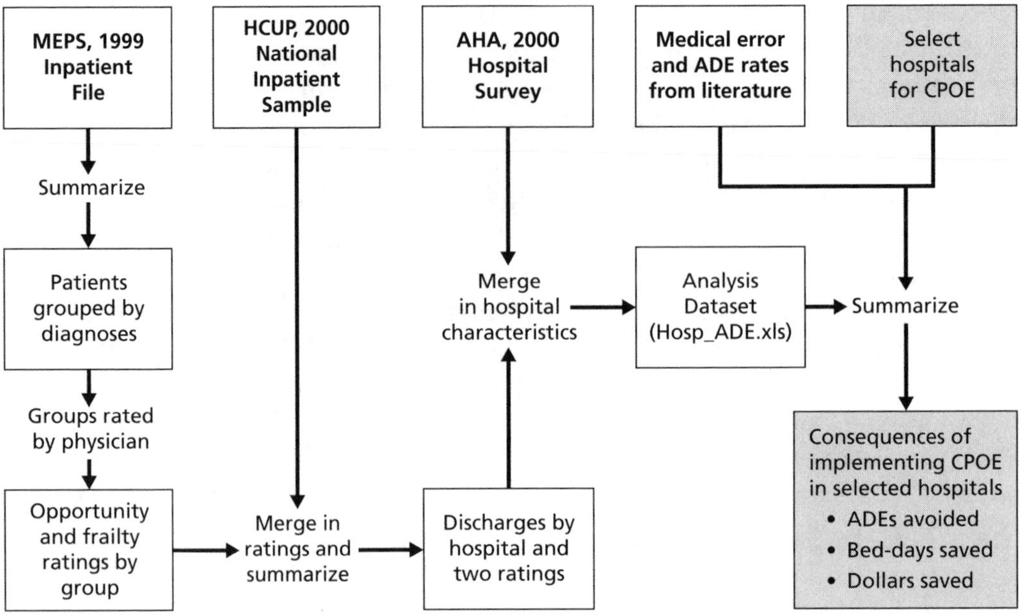

RAND *MG408-4.1*

In general, high ratings were given to human immunodeficiency virus (HIV), coagulation disorders, and renal failure. Medium or high ratings were given to cancers, pneumonia, cardiac disorders, diabetes, and liver disorders. We intended the frailty score to reflect the relative likelihood that the error would generate an ADE. Each score could have values low, medium, or high. High frailty ratings were given to liver and kidney disorders, and to acute myocardial infarctions (AMIs). Psychiatric diagnoses and eye-related diagnoses received low ratings.

We distributed errors and ADEs only to patients with high scores. To capture the length-of-stay effect, we distributed errors and ADEs to high-scoring patients in proportion to patient-days (rather than to admissions).

In the end, however, we combined the two scores by taking the minimum. That is, both the opportunity and frailty scores had to be high for the diagnosis to receive an overall high score. The Excel file MERADE.xls (available at http://www.rand.org/publications/MG/MG408, and also on the compact disc (CD) included with printed copies of this monograph) shows the ratings we gave to various diagnoses and (in some cases) combinations of diagnoses.

The National Inpatient Sample (NIS)

We merged the opportunity and frailty scores into NIS_2000_10PCT_SAMPLE_A, a public-use file available from the Agency for Healthcare Research and Quality's

(AHRQ's) Healthcare Cost and Utilization Project (AHRQ NIS, 2000). This file contains about 745,000 records, each summarizing a hospital discharge. Each record contains the following:

- Patient demographic data (age, race, sex) and diagnostic data (a principal diagnosis and up to 14 additional diagnoses)
- Hospital identifier
- Hospital-stay characteristics (principal procedure and up to 14 additional procedures, length of stay, total charges, who is expected to pay)
- Disposition after discharge (routine discharge, transfer to a short-term hospital, transfer to another type of facility, home healthcare, against medical advice, died in hospital)
- Sample weights for estimating national totals (e.g., total discharges, discharges by patient age or by principal diagnosis, total patient-days).

We matched diagnoses in order to add our opportunity and frailty scores to the Nationwide Inpatient Survey (NIS) file.

Hospital Data

We have two sources of data on hospitals. The file NIS_2000_HOSPITAL is distributed along with the Healthcare Cost and Utilization Project (HCUP) National Inpatient Sample described above. It contains information about each of the 994 hospitals that contributed data to the 2000 NIS sample. The American Hospital Association (AHA) surveys the nation's hospitals every year, and its survey provides far more information about each hospital than the NIS file does. The 2000 AHA survey included data on 6,044 hospitals. The NIS hospital file contains the AHA hospital identifier. By merging the files on this variable, we were able to supplement the HCUP hospital data with the AHA data. As is usual when comparing data from different sources, though, the match is imperfect: Only 730 hospitals are in the combined file.

Each record in the combined file includes the following:

- hospital characteristics (e.g., number of inpatient beds, Metropolitan Statistical Area (MSA) size, teaching versus nonteaching, ownership and control, primary service)
- sample weights for estimating national totals (e.g., total hospitals, hospitals by size, total beds).

We merged the discharge data with the hospital data and created a relatively small dataset for subsequent analysis. We imported these summarized data into an

Excel file, Hosp_ADE.xls (available at http://www.rand.org/publications/ MG/MG408 and on the CD included with printed copies of this monograph).

Rates of Medication Errors and ADEs

Based on the Bates studies, the Leapfrog Group (Birkmeyer et al., 2000) assumes that there are 7.6 serious medication errors per 1,000 patient-days and that CPOE could reduce the incidence of such errors by 55 percent.

In the absence of CPOE, about half of the serious medication errors will result in ADEs. With CPOE, potential ADEs (serious errors that do not result in injury) are reduced more than actual ADEs are. Thus the proportion of serious medication errors that result in ADEs increases to 75 percent (Bates et al., 1998).

Finally, preventing one ADE reduces the number of patient-days in hospital by 4.6 and reduces hospital "costs" by $4,685 (Bates et al., 1997). We put "costs" in quotes because this number is computed from hospital charges, scaled by the proportion of charges actually collected. It is not clear that this procedure yields the amount of money the hospital saves if it prevents one ADE.

There are many articles estimating the effects of CPOE on medication errors and ADEs, but they are the work of only a handful of authors, notably David Bates and his colleagues in Boston (Brigham and Women's Hospital, Massachusetts General Hospital, and Harvard Medical School). This means that the data on effect sizes may not be nationally representative.

Estimating Selected Effects of Inpatient CPOE

We perform "what-if" analyses by combining various factors with the analysis dataset, then varying those factors to represent different policies. The model with which we made these calculations is implemented in the Excel file Hosp_ADE.xls. Some of the factors are the medication error rates and ADE rates quoted earlier. Other factors specify which hospitals implement CPOE. Figure 4.2 shows the results of installing CPOE only in large hospitals, for which we have varied the dividing line between large and small hospitals. We look at ADEs avoided, and bed-days and dollars saved. Clearly, most of the effects can be realized by installing CPOE only in hospitals with, say, 100 beds or more. But it is not enough to install CPOE only in the really large hospitals.

The effects of inpatient CPOE are not large, given that the total expenditures on hospital care were $486 billion in 2002 (CMS NHE) and the total savings of inpatient CPOE are almost $1 billion. A hospital with over 500 beds will save about $1 million per year, according to this analysis. Smaller hospitals save less, and indeed save somewhat less per bed. We have not estimated any other effects of CPOE, although the Leapfrog Group has suggested that even larger savings might accrue through medication substitution, reduced laboratory testing and imaging, increased

Figure 4.2
Annual National-Level Effects of Using CPOE to Avoid Inpatient ADEs

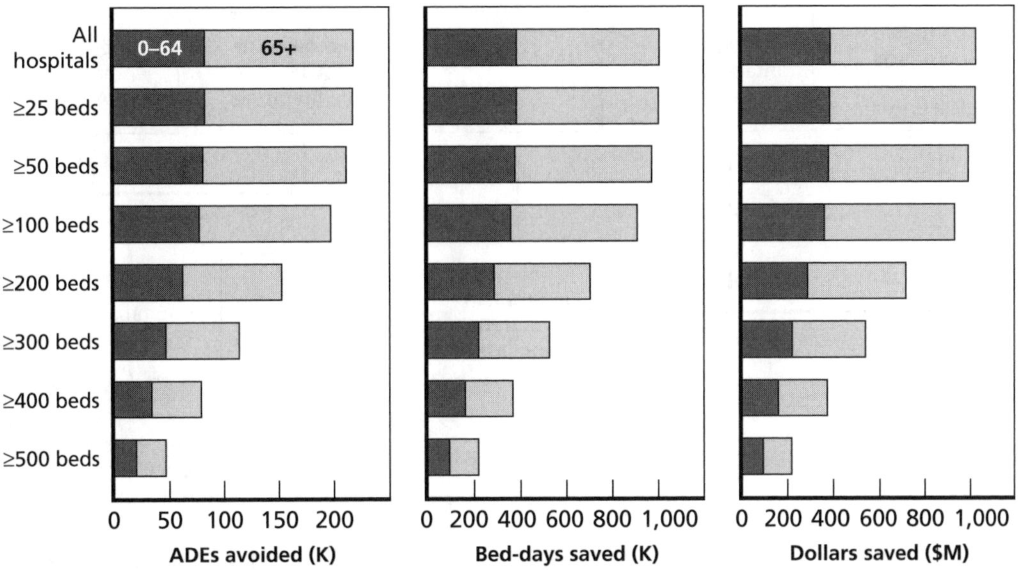

RAND *MG408-4.2*

use of clinical pathways, and gains in clinician efficiency (Birkmeyer et al., 2001). Indeed, Leapfrog argues that large hospitals but not small ones (they compare a 1,000-bed hospital with a 200-bed hospital) would find that adding a CPOE capability to an existing information infrastructure could pay for itself.

Figure 4.2 also splits the benefits according to whether the patient is under 65 or 65 and older, as an approximation to the Medicare population. Only about 13 percent of the population falls into the over-65 category, although this category accounts for more than its proportional share of hospital utilization (37 percent of hospital stays and 48 percent of hospital bed-days). But we calculated that about 62 percent of the benefits of inpatient CPOE would accrue to patients in the older group, because a higher fraction of patients 65 and older have diagnoses with high opportunity and frailty scores.[3]

The Ambulatory Setting

We used the process shown in Figure 4.3 to estimate the implications of these data for the nation. As before, data sources are listed across the top of the figure.

---

[3] With some effort, the reader can confirm this observation by accessing Hosp_ADE.xls and viewing the pivot table containing patient data (PivPatient).

Figure 4.3
Analysis Process for Estimating Effects of Ambulatory CPOE (ACPOE)

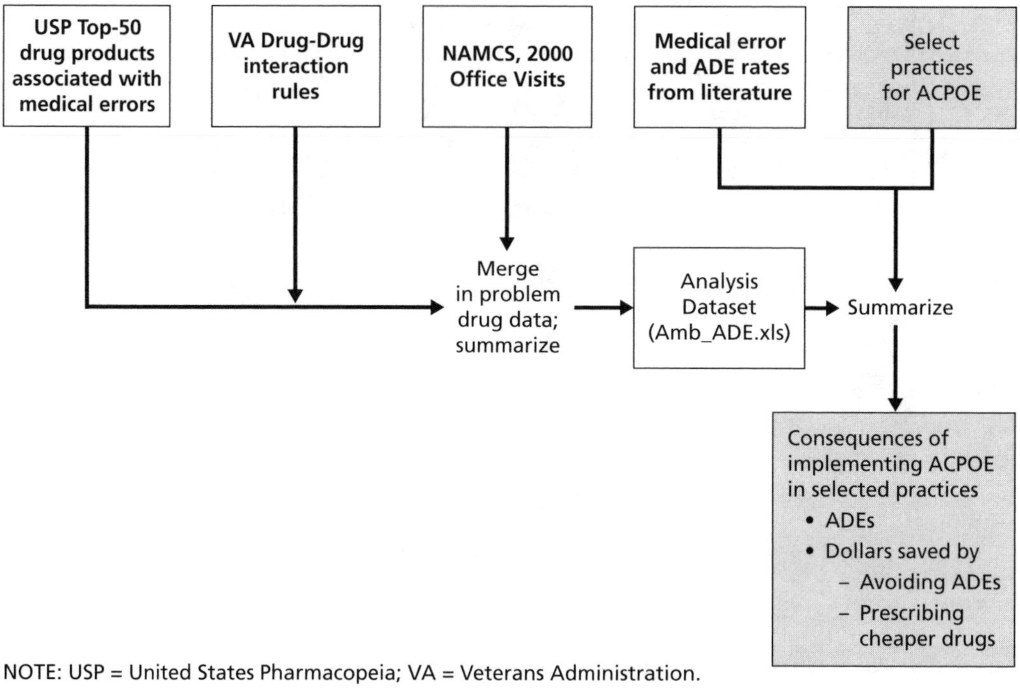

NOTE: USP = United States Pharmacopeia; VA = Veterans Administration.
RAND *MG408-4.3*

Drugs That Pose ADE Risks

In our model, we assumed an overall rate for serious medication errors and for ADEs, and we needed to devise a way to distribute the errors and ADEs among office visits with different characteristics. Descriptions of office visits came from the National Ambulatory Medical Care Survey (NAMCS), and the two kinds of NAMCS data elements that seem relevant for the purpose are "diagnoses" and "drugs ordered or provided."

We decided against using diagnoses as the basis for distributing ADEs over visits. Diagnoses in the NAMCS are not necessarily firm; indeed, the survey asks of each diagnosis whether it is "probable, questionable, or rule-out." Instead, we used the prescription drugs ordered or provided during the visit as the basis for deciding whether the visit was "eligible" for an ADE.

We used one list of problem drugs and a second list of pairs of drugs that interact. For the problem drugs, we used the top-50 drug products associated with medication errors that appear on the United States Pharmacopeia (USP) website. There were two original sources for interacting drug pairs. First, five of the top-50 drugs from the USP website were actually pairs. But most of our pairs came from Dr. Peter A. Glassman at the Los Angeles Veterans Administration (VA) Hospital (personal communication, 2003). He provided the pairs of drugs that triggered alerts in the VA CPOE, but he warned that there is no standard list, and there is much debate about how to choose interactions appropriately for CPOE (Glassman et al., 2002; Peng et al., 2003). These lists can be found in the Excel file RiskyDrugs.xls (available at www.rand.org/publications/MG/MG408 and on the CD included with printed copies of this monograph).

Some translation of the original lists was needed to make the names match drug names used in the NAMCS.

The National Ambulatory Medical Care Survey

As mentioned above, we obtained data on office visits to physicians from the NAMCS file for 2000. The NAMCS contains a sample of office visits to physicians. Each record (i.e., each visit) contains the following:

- Patient demographic data (age, sex, race)
- Characteristics of the practice (type of setting, whether a solo practice, who owns the office)
- Physician specialty
- Visit characteristics (examinations done, tests done, imaging done, diagnostic or screening services performed)
- Characteristics of medications ordered or provided during the visit (medication name, whether from a formulary)
- Sample weight for estimating national totals (e.g., total visits, total visits by specialty, total prescriptions).

We merged in the data on which drugs and drug combinations were most closely associated with medication errors to identify visits most likely to give rise to ADEs. We found that a problem drug or drug combination is ordered in about 18.3 percent of visits.

Rates of Medication Errors and ADEs

Medication errors and ADEs in ambulatory settings have been studied much less than in hospitals. The most comprehensive study of ambulatory ADEs appears to be the report by the Center for Information Technology Leadership (CITL), and we take several factors used in our model from that study (Johnston et al., 2003):

- 0.0098 ADE occurs per office visit
- 38 percent of ADEs are preventable
- 76 percent of preventable ADEs are avoided with a high-end CPOE.

To estimate the dollar savings that result from avoiding an ADE, we combine data from Johnston et al. and Jha et al. (2001). Johnston et al. state that 9.1 percent of preventable ADEs requires a hospitalization (if they are not prevented, of course), and Jha et al. report that the average cost is $10,376 for each such hospitalization. This information yields a cost of $944 per ADE for hospitalizations alone.

To estimate other costs, such as ER visits, follow-up office visits, and additional drugs, we turn to Johnson and Bootman (1995). They examined all drug-related morbidity, not just preventable ADEs, and estimated that the total healthcare costs of these events were $76.56 billion per year, of which $47.45 billion went for hospital care. If we inflate the $944 figure accordingly, we find a total savings of $1,600 from avoiding one ADE.

We included another source of savings in our model: substituting lower-priced drugs for higher-priced drugs. We took the total reduction to be 15 percent (Wang et al., 2003) of the expenditures on prescription drugs ($141 billion in 2001) (CMS NHE). The total savings from switching to cheaper drugs is over $20 billion.[4] The model distributes this savings over those drug mentions that the NAMCS reports are not from formularies.

As for inpatient CPOE, the data for effect sizes of ambulatory CPOE are from a handful of authors. They may not be nationally representative.

Estimating Effects of Ambulatory CPOE

We summarized the resulting merged file by a number of provider characteristics (e.g., practice size and specialty) to produce an analysis file. As with the inpatient file, this, too, is small enough to fit in an Excel spreadsheet and rich enough to support many "what-if" explorations. The Excel file, Amb_ADE.xls, is available at http://www.rand.org/publications/MG/MG408 and on the CD included with printed copies of this monograph.

As before, the "what-if" analysis consists of combining various factors with the analysis dataset, then varying those factors to represent different policies. Some of the factors are the ADE rates quoted above. Other factors specify which practices implement Ambulatory Computerized Physician Order Entry (ACPOE). Figure 4.4 shows the results of installing CPOE by practice size and ownership, which one might view as a proxy for the ability to afford a CPOE-capable Health Information Technology (HIT) system. We look at ADEs avoided and dollars saved due to avoided ADEs. National savings from avoiding outpatient ADEs are around $3.5 billion. Savings from substituting lower-priced drugs for higher-priced drugs (labeled "potential formulary savings" in the figure) total over $20 billion.

---

[4] Physicians may prescribe cheaper drugs because a HIT system displays them as alternatives to a more costly drug. But other measures—e.g., pricing policies—can promote switching from brand-name drugs to cheaper generics.

Figure 4.4
Annual National-Level Effects of Implementing Ambulatory CPOE in Physicians' Offices

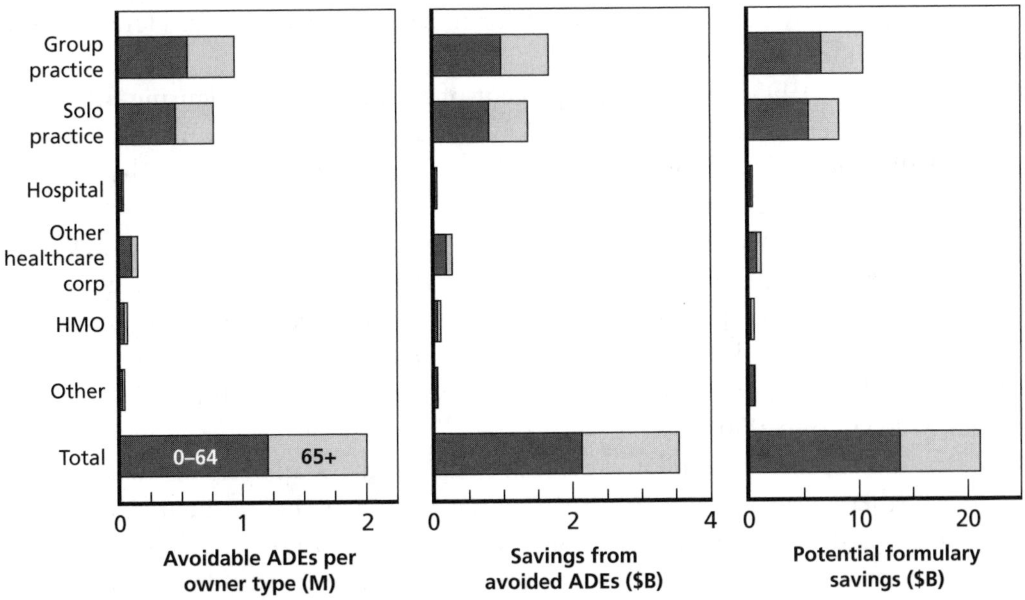

NOTE: HMO = health maintenance organization.
RAND *MG408-4.4*

Unlike for hospital-based CPOE, small practices cannot be overlooked. About 37 percent of the potential savings comes from solo practices. The question is, Can those practices afford ambulatory CPOE? Also, some group practices will have only two or three physicians, and they, too, may have trouble affording ambulatory CPOE. Wang et al. lay out a 5-year projection of costs and benefits of ambulatory CPOE, concluding that investing in such a system would pay off. Unfortunately, all the calculations are on a per-provider basis, and there is no discussion of whether the number of physicians in the practice would make a difference. We suspect that it would.

Patients 65 and older account for about 40 percent of ADEs, but only 35 percent of savings comes from cheaper drugs. Office visits by the elderly are more likely to be associated with medication errors, either because their drugs are more likely to be in USP's top-50 list or because they are more likely to be prescribed multiple drugs from the VA list that have interactions.

Mortality Due to Adverse Drug Events

We did not attempt to estimate mortality in our model. It is highly uncertain how many deaths due to ADEs could be avoided by use of CPOE. But we found support in the literature for 20,000 deaths per year from ADEs that occur in hospitals and a total of 106,000 deaths per year from ADEs that occur anywhere (both ambulatory and in hospitals). We also found support for much smaller numbers. Here is a sampling of the evidence.

Bates et al. (1995) found that 1 percent of ADEs are fatal. Figuring 6.5 ADEs per 100 nonobstetrical admissions and 30 million nonobstetrical admissions per year, we get 1.95 million ADEs, of which 19,500 are fatal. Bates et al. claim that none of the fatal ADEs was preventable.

Classen et al. (1997) found that 2.43 percent of hospital admissions was complicated by ADEs. The mortality rates of admits with ADEs and matched controls without ADEs were 3.5 percent and 1.05 percent, respectively. Omitting obstetrical admits (as Bates et al. do), we calculated 729,000 admits complicated by ADEs, of which 25,500 die. But 7,700 matched controls would die as well, bringing the excess mortality down to 18,000 per year.

Lazarou, Pomeranz, and Corey (1998) did a meta-analysis of adverse drug reactions (their term for adverse drug events) in which they estimated that such reactions caused 106,000 deaths (range: 76,000 to 137,000). They included both ADEs that occurred in the hospital and those that occurred outside and caused the admission to the hospital. Some fraction of the deaths from nonhospital ADEs could presumably be avoided by use of ambulatory CPOE.

Johnston et al. (2004) claim that ACPOE will avert more than 2 million ADEs and more than 190,000 hospitalizations per year. Using Classen et al.'s figure of 3.5 percent for the mortality among people hospitalized for ADEs, we estimated 6,650 fewer deaths from ambulatory ADEs.

The IOM report *To Err Is Human* (Corrigan and Donaldson, eds., 1999, p. 2) offers perhaps the lowest estimate; it says that "medication errors alone, occurring either in or out of the hospital, are estimated to account for over 7,000 deaths annually."

Estimating Savings from Reduced Laboratory and Radiology Utilization

Wang et al. (2003) report other savings as well, including

- a 15-percent reduction in drug costs due to substituting lower-priced drugs for higher-priced ones
- a 9-percent reduction in laboratory utilization
- a 14-percent reduction in radiology utilization.

From the *1997 Economic Census* (U.S. Census Bureau, 1997), we found that providers of ambulatory health care services (North American Industrial Classification System [NAICS]=621xxx) had receipts of $41 billion for laboratory services and diagnostic radiology. The *Economic Census* does not break out hospital receipts for these services, but the Healthcare Cost and Reporting Information System (HCRIS) gives us costs for a laboratory cost center ($15 billion) and for a diagnostic radiology cost center ($14 billion), both in 1999 (CMS HCRIS).

To bring the *Economic Census* numbers to a 1999 basis, we inflated them by 12 percent, which is the percentage increase in the NHE top line from 1997 to 1999. Our estimate of laboratory and diagnostic radiology services by providers of ambulatory care is thus $46 billion. Adding this amount to the hospital costs for the same services yields a total cost of $75 billion in 1999, which is equally divided between laboratory tests and diagnostic radiology procedures.

This total needs to be adjusted for double-counting. The patient's insurer or health plan is billed directly for some laboratory tests and diagnostic radiology procedures, but providers (e.g., hospitals or physician groups) pay for others themselves, then include a charge for the service in their own bills. The direct payments are counted once in the total, but the services originally paid for by providers are counted twice, once as revenue to the facility that performed the service and a second time as reimbursement of the amount the provider originally paid.

The Census Bureau conducts a Service Annual Survey (U.S. Census SAS) that provides sources of revenue for medical and diagnostic laboratories (NAICS=6215xx), among other things. From this source, we found that, in 1999, about 74 percent of patient-care revenue came directly from individuals and insurers. Applying the 74-percent factor to the above total yields an adjusted (i.e., purged of double-counting) total of $55.5 billion in expenditures on laboratory tests and diagnostic radiology. We assumed that this amount is equally divided between laboratory tests and diagnostic radiology procedures. Using the Wang et al. data, we estimated that potential savings on laboratory tests is $2.5 billion (9 percent of half of $55.5 billion) and $3.9 billion on diagnostic radiology procedures (14 percent of half of $55.5 billion), for a total of $6.4 billion in 1999.

Inflating Savings to Future Years

As described in Chapter Three, we have devised factors to inflate our estimates of changes in year 2000 expenditures to future years (see Tables 3.21 and 3.23).[5] Table

---

[5] In Chapter Three, we also developed a factor to adjust MEPS-based expenditure estimates for the year 2000 for differences between the MEPS and the NHE. It is not appropriate to apply this factor to the year 2000 savings estimated in this chapter, because we did not estimate these savings from expenditures reported in the MEPS.

4.1 shows the results. We inflated savings from avoiding inpatient ADEs with the hospital cost factors from Tables 3.21 and 3.23; the savings from avoiding ambulatory ADEs and reducing laboratory and radiology utilization with the physician factors; and the savings from prescribing drugs as much as possible from a formulary by the prescription drug factors. In the later years, the formulary savings dwarf the other savings, because the Centers for Medicare and Medicaid Services has estimated that expenditures on prescription drugs will rise at nearly 10 percent per year, much more quickly than any other component of healthcare expenditures. Because we estimate formulary savings as a percentage of expenditures on prescription drugs, the savings, too, rise at nearly 10 percent per year..

Table 4.1
CPOE-Mediated Savings ($billions) Inflated to Future Years

Year	Inpatient ADE Avoidance	Ambulatory ADE Avoidance	Formulary Savings	Reduced Lab and Radiology
2000	1.11	3.73	21.09	6.40
2005	1.57	5.29	40.53	9.08
2010	2.13	7.46	68.83	12.79
2015	2.80	10.21	107.98	17.52
2020	3.70	13.99	169.45	24.01

CHAPTER FIVE
Short-Term Effects of Preventive Services

James H. Bigelow, Ph.D., and Constance Fung, M.D.

Introduction

Here, we discuss our estimates of the short-term costs and benefits of influenza and pneumococcal vaccination, and of screening for cancers of the breast, cervix, and colon. These preventive services are among those recommended by the United States Preventive Services Task Force (USPSTF), a body that "provides evidence-based scientific reviews of preventive health services for use in primary care clinical settings, including screening, counseling, and chemoprevention" (Berg and Allen, 2001). *Screening* covers tests for early detection of many conditions, including breast, cervix, and colon cancers, hypertension, and hyperlipidemia. Counseling is recommended for appropriate persons on topics such as tobacco use, diet, and weight loss. *Chemoprevention* includes immunizations and prophylactic use of medications (e.g., aspirin for primary prevention of cardiovascular events). We did not estimate short-term effects of any counseling services, because we feel that their effects occur largely in the long term. We address the long-term effects in Chapter Seven.

Table 5.1 summarizes our results for the five preventive services we examined. Greater detail can be found in the five spreadsheets we constructed for calculating these results, which are available at http://www.rand.org/publications/MG/MG408 and on the compact disc (CD) included with printed copies of this monograph:

- Influenza.xls
- Pneumovax.xls
- CAbreast.xls
- CAcervix.xls
- CAcolon.xls.

These results assume that everybody for whom the USPSTF recommends these services receives these services. This is far from true today, as seen in the table. As

Table 5.1
Summary Results for Five Preventive Services (assumes 100-percent participation)

	Influenza Vaccination	Pneumococcal Vaccination	Screening for Breast Cancer	Screening for Cervical Cancer	Screening for Colorectal Cancer
Program Description					
Target Population	65 and older	65 and older	Women 40 and older	Women 18–64	50 and older
Frequency	1/yr	1/lifetime	0.5-1/yr	0.33-1/yr	0.1-0.2/yr
Population Not Currently Compliant	13.2 M	17.4 M backlog; 2.1 M new persons/yr	18.9 M	13 M	52 M
Financial Impacts					
Program Cost (with 100% compliance)	$134 M to $327 M/yr	$90 M/yr	$1,000 M to $3,000 M/yr	$152 M to $456 M/yr	$1,700 M to $7,200 M/yr
Financial Benefits	$32 M to $72 M/yr	$500 M to $1,000 M/yr	$0 to $643 M/yr	$52 M to $160 M/yr	$1,160 M to $1,770 M/yr
Health Benefits					
Reduced Workdays Missed	180,000 to 325,000/yr	100,000 to 200,000/yr			
Reduced Days Abed	1.0 M to 1.8 M/yr	1.5 M to 3.0 M/yr			
Deaths Avoided	5,200 to 11,700/yr	15,000 to 27,000/yr	2,200 to 6,600/yr	533/yr	17,000 to 38,000/yr
Years of Life Gained				13,000/yr	138,000/yr

we argue below, participation cannot be improved much without HIT to identify persons due for a preventive service and remind both doctor and patient.

The real benefits of these preventive services are the health benefits: They all reduce mortality rates, and the vaccination programs reduce days missed from work and days spent sick in bed. On purely financial grounds (financial benefits less program costs), only pneumococcal vaccination pays off. The other programs do no better than break even. However, in the worst case, their net costs are not very large. The pneumococcal vaccination program generates a net financial benefit because each person needs only one vaccination after age 65 and enjoys a reduced risk of pneumococcal diseases for the remainder of his or her life. The other programs require the preventive service to be repeated regularly.

We repeat that the figures in Table 5.1 are based on 100 percent of the eligible population receiving each service. At present, physicians deliver chemoprophylactic and screening preventive services only about half the time they should. McGlynn et al. (2003) looked at 439 indicators of healthcare quality, including many indicators for preventive services. Each indicator had the form "if the patient meets condition *X,* then the patient ought to receive service *Y.*" For example, "If a patient has diabetes, then he should receive an HbA1c (glycosylated hemoglobin) test every six months." Panels of experts developed the indicators, and no indicator that encountered significant disagreement was used in the study. Thus, if physicians are practicing medicine as they themselves believe they should, they ought to score a "Yes" on every indicator on just about every occasion it comes up. Instead, they score a "Yes" only 55 percent of the time.

The Absence of HIT Limits Participation

We argue that a lack of Health Information Technology (HIT) is a major barrier to raising this score, as the following example illustrates. Suppose, for example, that you are one of six physicians in a group, with a total of 12,000 patients. You have read the McGlynn et al. paper, and you wonder how well your practice is doing. Of course, you're pretty sure you are an exception—your practice is probably up around the 90-percent mark—but you'd like to check.

So you pick one recommendation, and you try to estimate how well your practice adheres to it. Let's take the recommendation that every person with diabetes should have an HbA1c test every six months, and the result of the test should be below some threshold (typically, 7 percent). (HbA1c is an indicator of long-term average blood glucose levels. If it is below the threshold, then the patient's blood glucose is generally under good control, although there may be short-term peaks and valleys that this test will not detect.) About 4.4 percent of adults are diagnosed with diabetes (another 2 percent of adults are thought to have undiagnosed diabetes), so your group should have about 528 diabetic patients.

But your group has paper records. To develop the two measures—the fraction of diabetics with an HbA1c test in the past six months, and the fraction of those tests with a result below the threshold—you must assign somebody to go through your paper records. Even if you maintain a list of all your diabetic patients (the first step toward a patient registry), that person must scan 528 records each time you want him or her to develop the measures. If he takes only one minute per record—to retrieve it, find the data he needs or verify that the data are not there, and refile the record—he will require 528 minutes, or almost 9 hours to develop the measures once.

It is not unreasonable to develop the measures once a month. Nor is it unreasonable to want to track another 50 or more measures (the McGlynn et al. paper looked at 439 indicators—153 for acute care, 248 for chronic care, and 38 for preventive care), each of which will take more or less the same amount of time to calculate. Clearly, it is out of the question to track very many quality measures in your paper-based group practice.

But can you not improve your adherence to care recommendations by having your nurse look over a patient's record when the patient has scheduled a visit? Doing so reduces the workload compared with developing the measures once a month, because the average patient will not visit that often. But it adds an appreciable fraction of a person-hour to the time the nurse devotes to that visit. And it fails to identify patients who are overdue for a service because they have not scheduled a visit.

The Presence of HIT Enables Greater Participation

Suppose you install an Electronic Medical Record System (EMR-S). At the core of the EMR-S is a database containing all the visits, tests, procedures, and prescriptions that you have ordered for every patient. It contains the patient's diagnoses and problem list. It is a matter of constructing and running a simple query (in a language such as structured query language [SQL]) to develop the HbA1c measures described above (among others). Each measure can be generated in a fraction of a second, as often as you desire. Moreover, the EMR-S can flag the services recommended for a patient each time the patient visits, with no increase in the time you or your nurse spends reviewing the patient's records. If you wish, the EMR-S can generate messages to send to patients overdue for services.

The bottom line is, with an EMR-S for which queries can be automated, you can track as many quality measures as you wish and use them to help improve your practice. Without an EMR-S for which queries can be automated, it is a major undertaking to track even a handful of quality measures, and you just cannot know readily how well you practice medicine. That is why you are able to tell yourself that your practice is up around the 90-percent mark in complying with McGlynn et al.'s quality indicators. Until you get an EMR-S, neither you nor anybody else will be able to test your claim.

There is, of course, no guarantee that a physician will use his or her EMR-S in this way. Most new users of information technology will try to adapt the technology to suit their existing work practices. At present, identifying patients due for preventive services is an existing practice of only a few physicians. Over time, however, more and more physicians will change their practices to take advantage of the technology.

The Impact of HIT on Compliance

A number of articles describe efforts to use information technology to improve physician compliance with recommended care (e.g., see Balas et al., 2000; Demakis et al., 2000; McDonald, Hui, and Tierney, 1992; Shea, DuMouchel, and Bahamonde, 1996). They all show that reminders improve physician compliance with recommended care, but only modestly. For example, compliance might rise from 50 to 60 percent.

It does not appear that any of these studies of reminders fed back the compliance scores to the participating physicians. There is some reason to believe that doing so would enhance the effectiveness of reminders, especially if each physician could see how his or her performance compared to his or her colleagues'.

It also does not appear that efforts were made to discover what prevented compliance from jumping to 90 percent or more, nor were efforts made to redesign the patient encounter so that higher compliance occurred as a matter of course.

Plan for the Remainder of the Chapter

In the rest of this chapter, we describe the analyses that led to the results in Table 5.1. We cover each preventive service in one section. In each section, we assume that all eligible persons receive the service, and we do not discuss further how HIT or anything else might help make this happen. These results, therefore, serve as bounds on the possible net benefits of these five preventive services, and not as projections of the net benefits of any particular program, HIT-enabled or not, for delivering these services.

Influenza Vaccination

Population

The USPSTF recommends an annual influenza vaccination for people 65 and over and for selected vulnerable populations (USPSTF, 1996). Even though the Centers for Disease Control and Prevention (CDC) has extended the recommendation to 50- to 64-year-olds (CDC, 2000), we will consider only the over-65 population in this analysis. Table 5.2 shows the size of a program to vaccinate all over-65s who do not currently receive vaccinations. Column 2 shows the over-65 population estimated from our Medical Expenditure Panel Survey (MEPS) file, broken out into three age categories. The percentage of over-65s that had a flu shot in the past year doubled, from 31 percent in 1989 to 64.5 percent in 2000 (NCHS, 2003). Columns 3 and 4 use this percentage to split the numbers in column 2 into currently vaccinated and currently unvaccinated populations.

Costs

Table 5.3 shows the cost of a program to vaccinate all over-65s who do not currently receive vaccinations. Column 2 repeats the number of people currently unvaccinated from Table 5.2. Column 3 provides an estimate of the cost of vaccinating all the

Table 5.2
Size of a Comprehensive Influenza Vaccination Program

Age Category	2000 Population from MEPS		
	Total	Currently Vaccinated	Currently Unvaccinated
65–74	18,965,229	12,232,573	6,732,656
75–84	13,379,824	8,629,986	4,749,838
85+	4,923,422	3,175,607	1,747,815
Total	37,268,474	24,038,166	13,230,308

unvaccinated people, at a price of $24.70 per vaccination (Bridges et al., 2000), which includes the cost of the vaccine itself, plus the cost of a nurse's time to administer the dose. This cost may be an overestimate. Medicare currently reimburses flu vaccinations at $10.10 per dose (CMS, 2004). We found a notice on the Internet[1] that quoted prices of about $9 per dose. If a nurse earning $40–$45,000 per year spends two minutes administering each dose, we must add another dollar to the cost. Thus, the final column estimates the cost of vaccinating the entire unvaccinated population at the Medicare reimbursement rate.

Benefits

The people who would have benefited from vaccination are those who were not vaccinated and got the flu. We extracted from the MEPS files all data for respondents with an influenza diagnosis, which we took to be the Clinical Classification Code–International Classification of Diseases, Revision 9 (CCC–ICD-9) pair in Table 5.4.

From our MEPS dataset, we estimated that about 15.6 million people report that they have the flu, of whom 1.2 million are 65 or over. Of those who report flu, 4.8 million people (0.5 million over 65) have a medical event that involves a flu diagnosis (mostly office visits and prescriptions). We have found no other source with which to compare these figures.

---

[1] See http://www.purchasing.wustl.edu; downloaded December 29, 2004.

Table 5.3
Cost of a Comprehensive Influenza Vaccination Program

Age Category	Currently Unvaccinated	Incremental Cost	
		$24.70/dose	$10.10/dose
65–74	6,732,656	$166 M	$68 M
75–84	4,749,838	$117 M	$48 M
85+	1,747,815	$43 M	$18 M
Total	13,230,308	$327 M	$134 M

Table 5.4
MEPS Diagnoses Included in Influenza

CCC	CCC Label	ICD9.3	ICD9.3 Label
123	Influenza	487	INFLUENZA*

NOTE: The asterisk is part of the ICD9.3 label. It does not refer to this note.

Influenza vaccination reduces the likelihood that the recipient will contract the disease. The benefits of this effect that we would like to estimate—or at least bound—are reductions in the following:

- Health care utilization
- Health care expenditures
- Days lost from work
- Days spent in bed
- Deaths.

Certain types of events reported in the MEPS have diagnoses associated with them: inpatient hospital stays, visits to hospital outpatient or emergency departments, office visits, and purchases of prescription drugs. Table 5.5 shows counts of events (i.e., utilization) and expenditures associated with an influenza diagnosis. We count expenditures on drugs prescribed for flu, but we do not include over-the-counter medications, since they are not reported in the MEPS.

The MEPS data are less helpful for estimating days lost from work or days spent sick in bed. These quantities are reported in the MEPS, but they are not allocated across specific conditions. Table 5.5 shows the total days lost and in bed per year by respondents who reported having the flu, including those who did not receive medi-

Table 5.5
Influenza-Related Healthcare Utilization and Expenditures, and Days Affected for Over-65s with Influenza[a]

Population	1,220,641
Utilization Measures	
Inpatient Stays	12,903[b]
Inpatient Nights	32,526[b]
Hosp Outpatient + Emergency Room (ER) Visits	38,020
Office Visits	472,801
Expenditures ($millions)	
Hospital	$57.1[b]
Physician	$43.1
Rx	$18.4
Other	$4.6
Total	$123.1
Days Affected	
Total Days Abed	9,666,998
Workdays Lost	1,702,756

[a]The items in this table were estimated from 482 observations from the MEPS dataset. The Agency for Healthcare Research and Quality (AHRQ) declines to report estimates made from fewer than 100 observations.
[b]These items have relative standard errors larger than 30 percent.

cal care for the condition. But we must remember that not all of these days may have been due to influenza.

The Centers for Disease Control and Prevention (CDC, 2000) has estimated that, on average, there are about 20,000 excess deaths per year from influenza, and we suppose that 75 percent of these occurred to people 65 years and older. (From Table 3.14, this is the proportion of total deaths that occur to people 65 and over.) Only a few of these deaths will be attributed to influenza on the death certificate. For the others, the cause of death will be something else—heart failure, for example. These other conditions render the victims fragile enough for a bout of influenza to be fatal. In 2000, the National Center for Health Statistics (NCHS) reported only 1,765 deaths whose official cause was influenza (NCHS GMWK, n.d.). The 1918 epidemic notwithstanding, influenza does not generally kill people who are healthy.

Clearly, not all of the utilization, expenditures, days lost, or deaths from flu will be avoided. We know that the efficacy of the influenza vaccine is not 100 percent. When there is a close antigenic match between the vaccine and the currently circulating influenza virus, efficacy is 70 to 80 percent (USPSTF, 1996). When the match is not close, efficacy can be as low as 50 percent (Bridges et al., 2000). Some of the utilization and expenditures are for people who were vaccinated. If the efficacy is only 50 percent, then there will be nearly as many cases of flu in the vaccinated population as in the unvaccinated one; therefore, we should allocate only half of the expenditures to the unvaccinated population. And vaccinating them will save, at most, half of that half. Table 5.6 shows these calculations carried out for three different efficacies. Similar calculations can be carried out for any of the quantities in Table 5.5. Because some days lost or days sick may have been for reasons other than flu, the effectiveness of flu vaccination in reducing these days will be even lower than its effectiveness in reducing utilization or expenditures.

We can define a factor, equal to the ratio of potential savings to total expenditures from Table 5.6, and express this factor as a function of efficacy. This function has a very simple mathematical form:

$$\text{Fractional\_Savings} = \frac{\text{Efficacy} \times P_{un}}{P_{un} + (1 - \text{Efficacy}) \times P_{vac}} \tag{5.1}$$

Figure 5.1 shows a graph of this function. Note that the factor does not depend on whether we are estimating reductions in expenditures or utilization or days lost or deaths. We can use the same formula for them all. For example, if we think that a

Table 5.6
Low Efficacy Compromises Potential Savings from Influenza Vaccination

	Symbol	Formula	Result		
Efficacy	E		0.5	0.75	1.0
Populations					
Vaccinated	P_{vac}		24,038,166	24,038,166	24,038,166
Unvaccinated	P_{un}		13,230,308	13,230,308	13,230,308
Total Flu Pop	C_{tot}		1,220,641	1,220,641	1,220,641
Incidence	I	$C_{tot}/(P_{vac}*(1-E)+P_{un})$	0.048	0.063	0.092
Flu cases					
Vaccinated	C_{vac}	$I*P_{vac}*(1-E)$	581,043	381,266	0
Unvaccinated	C_{un}	$I*P_{un}$	639,598	839,375	1,220,641
Expenditures ($millions)					
Total	D_{tot}		$123	$123	$123
Vaccinated	D_{vac}	$D_{tot}=D_{tot}*C_{vac}/C_{tot}$	$59	$38	$0
Unvaccinated	D_{un}	$D_{tot}*C_{un}/C_{tot}$	$65	$85	$123
Potential Savings		$E*D_{un}$	$32	$64	$123

Figure 5.1
Fractional Savings Versus Efficacy for Influenza Vaccination

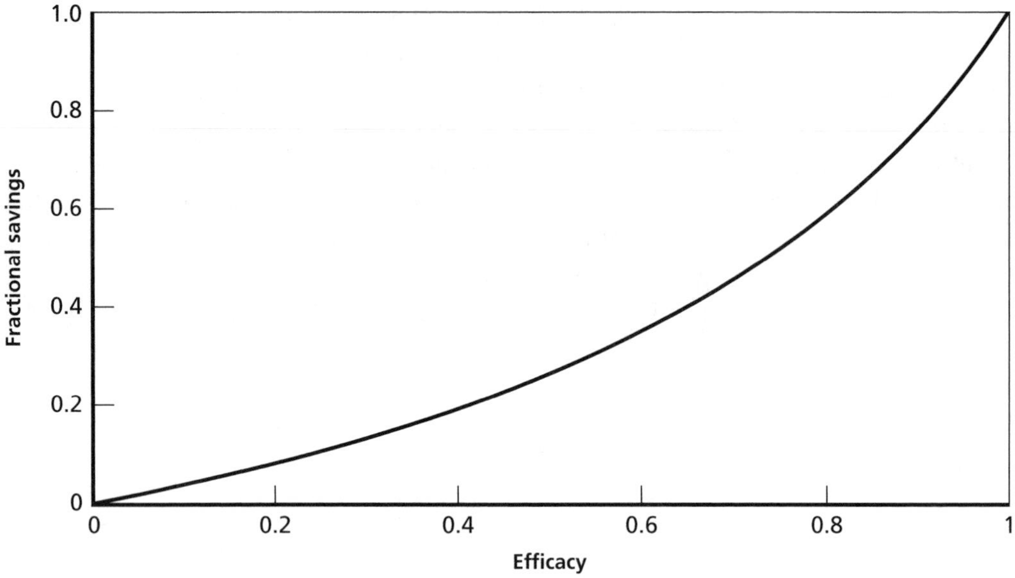

person who is vaccinated for influenza will experience only a 25-percent reduction in days sick in bed,[2] we calculated that a comprehensive influenza vaccine program will reduce this measure by only a little more than 10 percent.

Finally, we can easily consider a vaccination program that is less than comprehensive. If half the currently unvaccinated population is vaccinated, then we will estimate that both the costs and benefits of the program will be half those of the comprehensive program. On the cost side, this assumes that we cannot (or at least do not) identify segments of the population that are easy and inexpensive to recruit, and target them first. If the assumption is violated for cost, we should expect that a program that reaches half the currently unvaccinated population will cost *less than* half of the comprehensive program. On the benefit side, this assumes that we cannot (or again do not) target people affected more strongly than average by influenza. These would be people whose influenza-related utilization or expenditures are exceptionally high when they get the flu. If our assumption is violated for benefits, we should expect that a program that reaches half the currently unvaccinated population will produce *more than* half the benefits of the comprehensive program.

What, then, is the bottom line? To vaccinate everybody 65 and over will cost $134 million per year at Medicare reimbursement rates (Table 5.3). Even if the effi-

---

[2] We might arrive at this figure by arguing that the vaccine reduces the likelihood of influenza by 50 percent, but that only 50 percent of days spent sick in bed are due to influenza.

cacy is 100 percent, the total reduction in healthcare expenditures will be $123 million. Since the actual efficacy is 50 to 80 percent, the savings will lie between $32 million per year and $72 million per year. The program would break even in purely financial terms only if costs were low and the vaccine had an efficacy near 100 percent. With less-optimistic assumptions (higher costs or lower efficacy), there would be a net cost, not a net savings.

In many cost-benefit analyses, the investigator adds an amount for social benefits. Reductions in days lost from work, days spent sick in bed, and excess deaths (or years of life [life-years] lost) would be components of a social benefit. A reasonable value for a day lost from work might be $140, equivalent to an annual wage of around $30,000. Avoiding a day sick in bed, valued at the minimum wage, would be worth $50. We have argued that these flu deaths are deaths of fragile people, who probably would have died soon anyway. We assumed, then, that when we avoided a death through a flu vaccination, we added one or two years to a person's life. Valuing each year at $30,000,[3] or each avoided death at $45,000, we calculated the social benefits as set forth in Table 5.7.

As explained earlier in this chapter, only a fraction of these social benefits will actually be realized, depending on the efficacy of the vaccine and on the fractions of workdays lost and days sick in bed that were due to the flu. For example, if half the days lost and in bed were due to flu, and the efficacy of the vaccine is 50 to 80 percent, we save between 10.6 and 19.1 percent of those days. (Excess deaths are all due to flu, so they scale with efficacy in the same way as expenditures.) But even at the modest unit values we have assumed, it is relatively easy to generate a value for social benefits that exceeds the net financial costs.

Assignments of dollar values to social benefits are problematic in our view, however. We agree that social benefits are real, but with the possible exception of the value of workdays lost, they do not result in dollars in anybody's pocket. Hereafter, we present estimates of social benefits in their natural units only. We will not attempt to convert them into money.

---

[3] This is the same annual wage at which we valued days lost from work. Higher values per life-year (year of life gained) have been used in other sources—e.g., Tolley, Kenkel, and Fabian, eds. (1994) recommend a value per quality-adjusted life year between $70,000 and $175,000; however, even our lower number is enough to make an influenza vaccination program seem attractive.

Table 5.7
Potential Social Benefits of Comprehensive Influenza Vaccination

Benefit Category	Base Case	Unit Value	Extended Value
Workdays Lost	1,702,756	$140	$238 M
Days Sick Abed	9,666,998	$50	$483 M
Excess Deaths	20,000	$45,000	$900 M
Total			$1,621 M

Pneumococcal Vaccination

Population

The USPSTF recommends that people 65 and over receive a one-time pneumococcal vaccination.[4] Thus, the population to be vaccinated each year consists of the people who turn 65 during the year, plus a share of the people currently over 65 who are unvaccinated. From the MEPS, we found that approximately 2.1 million people per year turned 65 in 2000, and that there was a total of 37.3 million people over 65 (Table 5.2). The percentage of over-65s who have had a pneumococcal vaccination since age 65 climbed from 14.3 percent in 1989 to 53.2 percent in 2000 (NCHS, 2003), which yields a backlog of 17.4 million unvaccinated people over 65. In addition, about 2.11 million people turn 65 each year.

Costs

If we assume that a comprehensive pneumococcal program would eliminate that backlog over a 10-year period, then the program would have to perform 2.11 million vaccinations of people newly turned 65, plus 1.74 vaccinations from the backlog, or a total of about 3.85 million vaccinations per year.

The current Medicare reimbursement for a pneumococcal vaccination is $23.28 per dose (CMS, 2004). We therefore estimated the cost of the program to be $90 million per year.

Benefits

We wished to estimate the same benefits of pneumococcal vaccination that we did for influenza vaccination. We extracted from the MEPS files all data for respondents

---

[4] That is, they will not receive a second vaccination after age 65. They may have received a vaccination earlier, making the vaccination at age 65 their second.

with one of the diagnoses we included in our definition of the "pneumococcal" condition (Table 5.8).

According to the MEPS, 4.8 million people (1.4 million over 65) report at least one of these diagnoses in any year. Almost all of them receive care for the condition (4 million total; and 1.2 million over 65 have an event that lists one of these diagnoses). The National Institute of Allergies and Infectious Diseases (NIAID) quotes the following figures from CDC: 500,000 cases of pneumonia, 3,000 cases of meningitis, and 50,000 cases of bacteremia caused by *Streptococcus pneumoniae*.[5] But it is known that other organisms cause these diseases. The 5-digit ICD-9 code distinguishes among them, but the diagnoses in the MEPS does not. Indeed, the total cases reported by NIAID comprise 11.5 percent of the MEPS total.

Table 5.9 shows MEPS data on events associated with a pneumococcal diagnosis for people in the relevant age ranges. We counted expenditures on drugs prescribed for a pneumococcal infection, but could not include over-the-counter medications, because they are not reported in the MEPS.

It seems reasonable that these events would be the ones that pneumococcal vaccination would help people avoid. At first sight, therefore, over $6 billion is on the table. But pneumococcal vaccination will not avoid all of these events, because (1) other organisms will have caused some cases, and (2) the vaccine is not 100-percent effective at eliminating pneumococcal cases.

The days sick in bed or lost from work, and the deaths, are the quantities reported for people who have one of the diagnoses from Table 5.8. As with influenza vaccination, the MEPS data on outcomes are not allocated across medical conditions. Thus some—perhaps most—of these quantities might have nothing to do with those diagnoses, much less with cases caused by *Streptococcus pneumoniae*.

Table 5.8
MEPS Diagnoses Included in the "Pneumococcal" Condition

CCC	CCC Label	ICD9.3	ICD9.3 Label
002	Septicemia (except in labor)	038	SEPTICEMIA*
		790	ABNORMAL BLOOD FINDINGS*
076	Meningitis (except that caused by tuberculosis or sexually transmitted disease)	320	BACTERIAL MENINGITIS*
		322	MENINGITIS, UNSPECIFIED*
122	Pneumonia (except that caused by tuberculosis or sexually transmitted disease)	481	PNEUMOCOCCAL PNEUMONIA
		486	PNEUMONIA, ORGANISM NOS

NOTE: The asterisk is part of the ICD9.3 label. It does not refer to this note.
NOS = not otherwise specified.

---

[5] See http://www.niaid.nih.gov/factsheets/pneumonia.htm; accessed January 1, 2005.

We must adjust the numbers in Table 5.8 to account for this discrepancy. Figure 5.2 shows the fractional savings as a function of efficacy, using Equation (5.1). According to the CDC (1997), the effectiveness of the vaccine against invasive disease ranges from 56 to 81 percent, and *S. Pneumoniae* accounts for 25 to 35 percent of cases of community-acquired bacterial pneumonia in persons who require hospitalization. The overall effectiveness of pneumococcal vaccination against the diagnoses in Table 5.8 might be as low as 14 percent (25 percent of 56 percent) to as high as 28 percent (35 percent of 81 percent). From Figure 5.2, the corresponding range of savings is 7 to 15 percent. This fraction applies only after the entire unvaccinated population has been vaccinated. We assumed it would take 10 years to eliminate the backlog of unvaccinated people, and during that time the savings would be less. Still, after 10 years the annual savings would grow to from $500 million to $1 billion. This range exceeds the cost of the program, making a pneumococcal vaccination program a net money saver.

If we assume that half of the days spent in bed and workdays lost are due to the diagnoses in Table 5.8, then the overall effectiveness of the vaccination against these

Table 5.9
Pneumococcal-Related Healthcare Utilization and Expenditures, and Days Affected for Over-65s with a Pneumococcal Diagnosis[a]

Population	1,389,907
Utilization Measures	
Inpatient Stays	566,594
Inpatient Nights	4,505,541
Hosp Outpatient + ER Visits	305,089
Office Visits	1,540,672
Expenditures ($millions)	
Hospital	$5,579.9
Physician	$706.7
Rx	$76.8
Other	$24.8
Total	$6,388.2
Outcomes	
Total Days Abed	38,379,477
Workdays Lost	2,792,188
Deaths	158,285

[a]The items in this table were estimated from 517 observations from the MEPS dataset. The AHRQ declines to report estimates made from fewer than 100 observations. All estimates have relative standard errors smaller than 30 percent.

Figure 5.2
Fractional Savings Versus Efficacy for Pneumococcal Vaccination

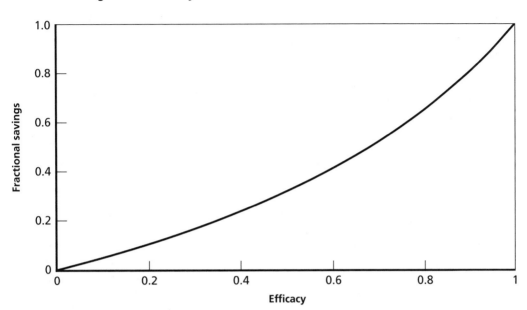

RAND *MG408-5.2*

outcomes will be half of the effectiveness against the events associated with the diagnoses, or between about 4 and 8 percent. Once everybody was vaccinated, annual days in bed should drop by 1.5 to 3 million and annual workdays lost should drop by 100,000 to 200,000. For comparison, all people 65 and older spent 377 million days in bed and lost 31 million workdays to sickness.

The CDC (1997) estimates that pneumococcal infection causes 40,000 deaths per year. Since these deaths are due to *S. pneumoniae,* we only need to adjust for the efficacy of the vaccine. Deaths should be reduced by 37 to 67 percent, or 15,000 to 27,000.[6] Most of the people who die of pneumonia are quite elderly (about half are 85 or older (CDC, 2003) and, typically, they have comorbidities. Thus, we should expect that each death avoided will translate into no more than one or two years of additional life.

---

[6] The 37- and 67-percent figures are the fractional savings from Figure 5.2 corresponding to efficacies of 56 and 81 percent, respectively.

Screening for Breast Cancer

Population

We considered a program that provides a screening mammogram for every woman over 40 every one to two years. The USPSTF does not recommend a program quite this lavish, as can be seen by this quote from its website:[7]

> The USPSTF found fair evidence that mammography screening every 12–33 months significantly reduces mortality from breast cancer. Evidence is strongest for women aged 50–69, the age group generally included in screening trials. For women aged 40–49, the evidence that screening mammography reduces mortality from breast cancer is weaker, and the absolute benefit of mammography is smaller, than it is for older women. Most, but not all, studies indicate a mortality benefit for women undergoing mammography at ages 40–49, but the delay in observed benefit in women younger than 50 makes it difficult to determine the incremental benefit of beginning screening at age 40 rather than at age 50.
>
> The absolute benefit is smaller because the incidence of breast cancer is lower among women in their 40s than it is among older women. The USPSTF concluded that the evidence is also generalizable to women aged 70 and older (who face a higher absolute risk for breast cancer) if their life expectancy is not compromised by comorbid disease. The absolute probability of benefits of regular mammography increase[s] along a continuum with age, whereas the likelihood of harms from screening (false-positive results and unnecessary anxiety, biopsies, and cost) diminish[es] from ages 40–70. The balance of benefits and potential harms, therefore, grows more favorable as women age. The precise age at which the potential benefits of mammography justify the possible harms is a subjective choice. The USPSTF did not find sufficient evidence to specify the optimal screening interval for women aged 40–49.

Using population estimates developed from the MEPS files and data on the fraction of women screened from *Health, United States* (NCHS, 2003), we calculated the additional population that a comprehensive breast cancer screening program would need to reach (Table 5.10).

Costs

We considered two comprehensive programs: one that screens every currently unscreened woman once per year and one that screens every woman once every two years. The results of a test will be abnormal with a probability that depends on the age of the woman (Salzmann, Kerlikowske, and Phillips, 1997) and, we assumed, is proportional to the interval between screenings. An abnormal result will trigger a

---

[7] See http://www.ahrq.gov/clinic/uspstf/uspsbrca.htm; accessed January 25, 2005.

Table 5.10
Female Populations Currently Screened and Unscreened for Breast Cancer

| Age Category | Percentage Screened | 2000 Female Population from MEPS | | |
		Total	Screened	Unscreened
40–44	64.20%	11,337,051	7,278,386	4,058,664
45–49	64.20%	9,053,382	5,812,271	3,241,111
50–54	78.60%	9,053,382	7,115,958	1,937,424
55–59	78.60%	6,018,850	4,730,816	1,288,034
60–64	78.60%	6,018,850	4,730,816	1,288,034
65–69	74.00%	5,176,293	3,830,457	1,345,836
70–74	74.00%	5,176,293	3,830,457	1,345,836
75–79	61.30%	3,982,187	2,441,081	1,541,106
80–85	61.30%	3,982,187	2,441,081	1,541,106
85+	61.30%	3,477,526	2,131,723	1,345,803
Total		63,276,000	44,343,046	18,932,954

workup to determine whether it is a false alarm or a cancer. Table 5.11 shows our calculation of the number of screening tests, workups, and cancers discovered for our two programs. The number of cancers actually discovered could be lower than the

Table 5.11
Annual Number Screened, Abnormal Tests, and Potential Cancers

| Age Category | Number Screened | | Abnormal Tests (1- or 2-year interval) | Potential Cancers (1- or 2-year interval) |
	1-year interval	2-year interval		
40–44	4,058,664	2,029,332	158,288	5,090
45–49	3,241,111	1,620,555	126,403	6,411
50–54	1,937,424	968,712	48,436	4,508
55–59	1,288,034	644,017	32,201	3,581
60–64	1,288,034	644,017	25,761	4,422
65–69	1,345,836	672,918	26,917	5,546
70–74	1,345,836	672,918	26,917	6,070
75–79	1,541,106	770,553	30,822	7,457
80–85	1,541,106	770,553	30,822	7,357
85+	1,345,803	672,901	26,916	6,425
Total	18,932,954	9,466,477	533,482	56,867

number in the table, if the test is imperfect. Because the test is repeated periodically, however, cancers missed by one test should be detected by a later test.

According to Salzmann, Kerlikowske, and Phillips (1997), a mammogram costs $106 ($46–$144) and working up an abnormal result costs $345 ($182–$509). Disregarding the cost of treating the cancers that are discovered, then, the program that screens annually will cost about $2 billion dollars per year ($1–$3 billion/year), and the program that screens once every two years will cost about half that amount.

Benefits

We wished to estimate the same benefits of breast cancer screening that we did for influenza vaccination. We extracted from the MEPS files all data for female respondents with any of the diagnoses in Table 5.12.[8]

We estimate from our MEPS dataset that approximately 1.1 million people (1 million over 40) report one or more of the above diagnoses. Almost all have at least one healthcare event (e.g., an office visit, a hospital stay, a prescription) that lists a diagnosis from Table 5.12. The American Cancer Society (2003a) estimates that 55,700 *in situ* cases and 211,300 invasive (regional and distant) cases were newly diagnosed in 2003. The prevalence from the MEPS is thus consistent with an average treatment time—or perhaps treatment plus follow-up—of about four years (1.1 million women in treatment at a point in time divided by 267,000 new cases per year). The relative 5-year survival rate is 87 percent overall, so clearly most women survive longer than four years.

We extracted from the MEPS files the utilization measures and expenditures for women 40 and older who have a breast cancer diagnosis, including only events with an associated diagnosis of breast cancer. These are the events that we might expect to be changed if all women were screened for breast cancer. Table 5.13 shows the results.

Table 5.12
MEPS Diagnoses Included in Breast Cancer

CCC	CCC Label	ICD9.3	ICD9.3 Label
024	Cancer of breast	174	MALIG NEO FEMALE BREAST*
		233	CA IN SITU BREAST-*/
		239	UNSPECIFIED NEOPLASM*
		V10	HX OF MALIGNANT NEOPLASM*

NOTE: The asterisk is part of the ICD9.3 label. It does not refer to this note.

---

[8] If it seems odd to include ICD9.3=239 (UNSPECIFIED NEOPLASM*) and V10 (HX OF MALIGNANT NEOPLASM*), remember that it takes a pair of codes (CCC=024 *and* an ICD9.3 code) to place a person in our breast cancer category.

Table 5.13
Utilization and Expenditures on Breast
Cancer–Related Events for Women over 40[a]

	Value
Population	998,503
Utilization Measures	
Inpatient Stays	156,185
Inpatient Nights	504,096[b]
Hosp Outpatient + ER Visits	1,305,645
Office Visits	3,751,912
Expenditures ($millions)	
Hospital	$3,410.6[b]
Physician	$994.5
Rx	$389.6
Other	$163.4
Total[a]	$4,958.1[b]

[a]The items in this table were estimated from 361 observations from the MEPS dataset. The AHRQ declines to report estimates made from fewer than 100 observations.
[b]These items have relative standard errors larger than 30 percent.

Of the about $5 billion in expenditures, how much might be saved? Salzmann, Kerlikowske, and Phillips (1997) show almost no difference in treatment cost between screened and unscreened women. If this is what we can expect from screening, there are no savings to be had.

By contrast, Kerlikowske et al. (1999) show that treatment of cancer *in situ* is about one-third less costly than treatment of regional cancer. Taplin et al. (1995) report that, during initial care (the first six months after diagnosis), the cost of all care for a woman with breast cancer *in situ* is one-third less than for a woman with regional breast cancer. Optimistically, we supposed that cancers diagnosed in screened women are all *in situ* and that cancers in unscreened women are regional, and calculated an upper bound on the savings from screening all women.

From Table 5.10, there are 63.3 million women over 40, 44.3 million of whom are screened and 18.9 million of whom are unscreened. If the average expenditure on breast cancer events per screened woman is two-thirds of the average expenditure per unscreened women, and if the total expenditure is $4.96 billion (from Table 5.13), then the expenditure per screened woman is $68 per year and per unscreened woman, $102 per year. Screening the 18.6 million women who are currently unscreened will save $34 per woman per year, or a total of $643 million. But remember, this is an upper bound, one that assumes cancers are never discovered *in situ* without screening and always discovered *in situ* with screening. Clearly, the savings is considerably smaller than the cost of the program.

The real benefit of breast cancer screening, then, lies in the health benefits. To the degree that screening identifies cases earlier, screening increases survival. According to the 2004 edition of CDC's "burden book" (CDC, 2004a): "Timely mammography screening among women aged 40 or older can prevent approximately 16% of all deaths from breast cancer . . . ." The same source reports 41,394 deaths from breast cancer in 2001. It is unclear whether this source means that the death rate among screened women is 16 percent lower than among unscreened women, or whether total deaths from breast cancer could be reduced by 16 percent if all women were screened. If they mean the former, one can calculate that comprehensive screening would reduce deaths from breast cancer by 2,238 per year. If they mean the latter, deaths would be reduced by 6,623 per year.

Screening for Cervical Cancer

Population

USPSTF (2003) recommends screening of women at least every three years, starting at age 21 or beginning of sexual activity and continuing to age 65. They recommend against screening for women 65 and older. We analyze a program that screens every female between 18 and 65. Using population estimates from the MEPS files and data on the fraction of women screened from *Health, United States* (NCHS, 2003), we calculated the additional population that a comprehensive cervical cancer screening program would need to reach (Table 5.14).

Table 5.14
Female Populations Currently Screened, Unscreened, and Recommended for Screening for Cervical Cancer

Age Category	Percentage Screened	Total	Screened	Unscreened	Recommended
18–49	85.20%	64,858,181	55,259,170	9,599,011	9,599,011
50–64	83.70%	21,091,082	17,653,235	3,437,846	3,437,846
65–74	71.60%	10,352,585	7,412,451	2,940,134	
75+	56.80%	11,441,901	6,499,000	4,942,901	
Total		107,743,749	86,823,856	20,919,892	13,036,857

Costs

Marle et al. (2002) report that the cost of a *Papanicolaou* (PAP) smear is $32. They assumed that 0.06 percent of screened women would receive a colposcopy and biopsy (cost, $485), after which no cancer would be found, and that 6.2 percent of women would receive an average of 1.8 repeat PAP smears, at a cost of $49. Thus, for each screening cycle, the program would cost about $35 per woman. To provide a PAP test once every three years to every unscreened woman that the USPSTF recommends receive one would cost $152 million per year. More-frequent screening would cost proportionately more (e.g., annual screening would cost $456 million per year).

Benefits

To estimate the same benefits of cervical cancer screening that we did for influenza vaccination, we extracted from the MEPS files all data for female respondents with any of the diagnoses in Table 5.15. Approximately 0.3 million women in the MEPS are between 18 and 64 and report one or more of these diagnoses.

We extracted from the MEPS files the utilization and expenditures for women between 18 and 64 who have a cervical cancer diagnosis, including only events with an associated diagnosis of cervical cancer. These are the events that we might expect to be changed if all women were screened for cervical cancer. Table 5.16 shows the results.

Of the about $400 million, we want to know how much might be saved. Marle et al. give costs for diagnosis and treatment for cancers at different stages: cervical intraepithelial neoplasia, $1,950; stage IA, $5,315; later stages, an average of $10,530. Assuming that the incidence of cervical cancers is the same in the screened and unscreened populations, we used these per-case costs to distribute the dollars, in Table 5.17.

Table 5.15
MEPS Diagnoses Included in Cervical Cancer

CCC	CCC Label	ICD9.3	ICD9.3 Label
026	Cancer of cervix	180	MALIG NEOPL CERVIX UTERI*
		233	CA IN SITU CERVIX UTERI
		239	UNSPECIFIED NEOPLASM*
		795	ABN PAP SMEAR-CERVIX-*/
		V10	HX OF MALIGNANT NEOPLASM*

NOTE: The asterisk is part of the ICD9.3 label. It does not refer to this note.

Table 5.16
Utilization and Expenditures on Cervical Cancer–Related Events for Women Between 18 and 64[a]

	Value
Population	315,828
Utilization Measures	
Inpatient Stays	23,662
Inpatient Nights	69,347
Hosp Outpatient + ER Visits	40,070
Office Visits	510,841
Expenditures ($millions)	
Hospital	$245.4
Physician	$146.3
Rx	$2.3
Other	$5.7
Total	$399.7

[a]The items in this table were estimated from 124 observations from the MEPS dataset. The AHRQ declines to report estimates made from fewer than 100 observations. All estimates have relative standard errors smaller than 30 percent.

Table 5.17
Calculation of Potential Savings from Comprehensive Cervical Cancer Screening

	Maximum Impact	Minimum Impact
Screened women in ages 18–64 (Table 5.14)	72.91 M	72.91 M
Unscreened women in ages 18–64 (Table 5.14)	13.04 M	13.04 M
Cost per screened case	$1,950	$5,315
Cost per unscreened case	$10,530	$10,530
Average cost per case	$3,252	$6,106
Total cases (total cost/average cost per case)	122,940	65,465
Cases among unscreened women (prorated)	18,648	9,930
Potential savings (unscreened cases × Δcost per case)	$160 M	$52 M

According to the American Cancer Society (2003b), about 12,200 new cases of cervical cancer appeared in 2003. Our estimated numbers of cases in Table 5.17 are much larger than this, but they may include women receiving follow-up services years after their cancers were first diagnosed. Women whose cancers are discovered at an early stage survive longer. And, because screening results in the discovery of cancers at an earlier stage, one should expect that a higher fraction of screened women would have cervical cancer–related events in the MEPS, which will tend to reduce the cost advantage of screening. But even ignoring this effect, a cervical cancer screening program can do no more than break even financially.

The real benefit of cervical cancer screening, then, lies in the health benefits. Marle et al.'s simulations estimate that, for a 3-year screening interval, 41 deaths will be prevented and 1,022 life-years gained per million women in the program per year. A comprehensive program will reach about 13 million women who are not currently screened (Table 5.14). Thus, it should prevent 533 deaths and gain 13,286 life-years. The reductions in deaths amount to 13 percent of the total deaths from cervical cancer (CDC, 2003). Since 85 percent of 18- to 64-year-old women are already being screened, a comprehensive program would require a 50-percent lower death rate among screened women to achieve this effect.

Screening for Colorectal Cancer

Population

The USPSTF (2002a) recommends that men and women 50 years and older be screened for colorectal cancer. Of people over 50, 66 percent reported having no sigmoidoscopy or colonoscopy in the past five years, and 79 percent reported no fecal occult blood test in the past year (CDC, 2002). According to the MEPS files, there were about 78 million people 50 years and older in 2000. We calculated that a comprehensive colorectal cancer screening program would need to reach an additional 52 million people.

Costs

The range of costs for the various screening procedures is wide, and each procedure has its own recommended frequency, as reported by Pignone et al. (2002) and listed in Table 5.18

A screening program should consist of a combination of tests—for example, an annual fecal occult blood test (FOBT) plus a colonoscopy every tenth year. The cost for this combination is between $32 and $139.20 per person per year, which translates to between $1.7 billion per year and $7.2 billion per year for a comprehensive program.

Benefits

To estimate the same benefits of colorectal cancer screening that we did for influenza vaccination, we extracted from the MEPS files all data for respondents with any of the diagnoses in Table 5.19. We estimated that approximately 0.35 million people over 50 report one or more of these diagnoses.

Table 5.18
Costs and Recommended Frequencies of Colorectal Cancer Screening Tests

Test	Minimum Cost	Maximum Cost	Recommended Frequency
Colonoscopy	$285.00	$1,012.00	Once in 10 years
Colonoscopy with Polypectomy	$434.00	$1,519.00	Once in 10 years
Sigmoidoscopy	$80.00	$400.00	Once in 5 years
Fecal Occult Blood Test (FOBT)	$3.50	$38.00	Annually

SOURCE: Pignone et al., 2002.

Table 5.19
MEPS Diagnoses Included in Colorectal Cancer

CCC	CCC Label	ICD9.3	ICD9.3 Label
014	Cancer of colon	153	MALIGNANT NEOPLASM COLON*
		159	OTH MALIG NEO GI/PERITON*
		199	MALIGNANT NEOPLASM NOS*
		V10	HX OF MALIGNANT NEOPLASM*
015	Cancer of rectum and anus	154	MALIG NEO RECTUM/ANUS*

NOTE: The asterisk is part of the ICD9.3 label. It does not refer to this note.
NOS = not otherwise specified.

We extracted from the MEPS files the utilization and expenditures for events associated with any of these diagnoses for all persons 50 and older. These are the events that might be changed by a screening program for colorectal cancer. Table 5.20 shows the results.

Over $2.8 billion are spent on these events. Even if all of that amount could be saved, the screening program would not break even. Data reported in Pignone et al. (2002) and in Taplin et al. (1995) suggest that the cost of treating colorectal cancer while it is still local is at least half the cost of treating the cancer after it has become regional or distant. We use this observation to allocate the $2.84 billion from Table 5.20 to the screened and unscreened populations in the same way as illustrated in Table 5.17 for breast cancer screening. This allocation suggests that comprehensive screening might save $1.13 billion per year.

We can compare this figure with a calculation based on Sonnenberg, Delco, and Inadomi (2000), who simulated a cohort of 100,000 people starting at age 50 and continuing until death. Total treatment costs for an unscreened population are $136 million. Total treatment costs for a population screened by colonoscopy every ten years are $34 million. If we assume that 50-year-olds live, on average, 30 more years, the savings in treatment costs will be $34 per person per year. We envision screening 52 million people, so every year should see a reduction of about $1.77

Table 5.20
Utilization and Expenditures on Colorectal
Cancer–Related Events for Persons 50 and Older[a]

	Value
Population	353,526
Utilization Measures	
Inpatient Stays	109,377
Inpatient Nights	1,771,930
Hosp Outpatient + ER Visits	298,938
Office Visits	1,069,678
Expenditures ($millions)	
Hospital	$2,176.2
Physician	$564.5
Rx	$13.0
Other	$0.0
Total	$2,842.7

[a]The items in this table were estimated from 150 observations from the MEPS dataset. The AHRQ declines to report estimates made from fewer than 100 observations. All estimates have relative standard errors smaller than 30 percent.

billion in treatment costs, which seems like pretty good agreement, given all the assumptions we made. We conclude that a screening program for colorectal cancer increases net healthcare expenditures, and so do Sonnenberg, Delco, and Inadomi.

The real benefit of colorectal cancer screening, then, lies in the health benefits. The 2004 burden book (CDC, 2004a, p. 23) states that

> [r]outine screening for colorectal cancer, as recommended by the U.S. Preventive Services Task Force, can reduce the number of people who die of this disease by at least 30%.

The same source (CDC, 2004, p. 56) also claims that

> Studies have found that people who had a sigmoidoscopy [had] 59% fewer deaths from colorectal cancers within reach of a sigmoidoscope than people who had not had a sigmoidoscopy.

Colorectal cancer causes about 57,000 deaths per year (CDC, 2003); a 30-percent reduction amounts to 17,100 deaths prevented annually. Assuming, instead, that screening reduces the death rate by 59 percent, we found that comprehensive screening should prevent 27,800 deaths, almost 50 percent of the total. Sonnenberg, Delco, and Inadomi assume that colonoscopy reduces mortality by 75 percent, which would imply that a comprehensive program would prevent 37,900 deaths per year.

Sonnenberg, Delco, and Inadomi's simulation also shows that comprehensive use of colonoscopy gains 7,952 life-years in a cohort of 100,000 people followed from age 50 to death. Assuming a life expectancy at age 50 of 30 years, we obtained a gain of 7,952 life-years per 3 million person-years in the screening program. Scaling this figure up to the 52 million people in our comprehensive program yields a gain of about 137,800 life-years per year.

CHAPTER SIX

Management of Chronic Diseases

James H. Bigelow, Ph.D., Kateryna Fonkych, and Constance Fung, M.D.

Introduction

According to the Disease Management Association of America (DMAA),[1] *disease management* is

> a system of coordinated healthcare interventions and communications for populations with conditions in which patient self-care efforts are significant. Disease management:
>
> - supports the physician or practitioner/patient relationship and plan of care,
>
> - emphasizes prevention of exacerbations and complications utilizing evidence-based practice guidelines and patient empowerment strategies, and
>
> - evaluates clinical, humanistic, and economic outcomes on an ongoing basis with the goal of improving overall health.

Disease Management *Components* include:

- Population Identification processes

- Evidence-based practice guidelines

- Collaborative practice models to include physician and support-service providers

- Patient self-management education (may include primary prevention, behavior modification programs, and compliance/surveillance)

---

[1] The DMAA website is http://www.dmaa.org/definition.html; accessed December 30, 2004.

- Process and outcomes measurement, evaluation, and management

- Routine reporting/feedback loop (may include communication with patient, physician, health plan and ancillary providers, and practice profiling)

Full Service Disease Management Programs must include all 6 components. Programs consisting of fewer components are Disease Management Support Services.

We have chosen four chronic diseases to analyze—diabetes, congestive heart failure (CHF), asthma, and chronic obstructive pulmonary disease (COPD)—because most studies of actual disease management programs deal with these four conditions. (There are, of course, many other chronic conditions that one might manage, including human immunodeficiency virus (HIV), cancer, arthritis, allergies, and depression.) These studies measure the effects of programs on the frequencies of hospitalizations and visits to the hospital emergency room in the short term (i.e., within the first year or two of a person's enrollment). A hospitalization is the signal that there has been an exacerbation or complication. We estimate the effects of disease management on healthcare utilization and cost, and on some measures of population health status. We embed our estimates of these effects in the world of 2000, which is the world described by the trajectory file we assembled from the Medical Expenditure Panel Survey (MEPS) (see Chapter Two). Thus, we assume the same population, the same technology, and the same propensities to seek medical attention that gave rise to our database. In short, we are asking what healthcare in 2000 might have looked like if everybody with one of the four chronic conditions we examined had been enrolled in a disease management program of the kind we describe below.

In the remainder of this section, we provide a generic discussion of the disease management programs we later analyze. We discuss program design and then the role of Health Information Technology (HIT). Then we outline our methods for estimating program costs and benefits. In the four subsequent sections, we estimate costs and benefits for the four chronic diseases we have chosen to analyze. Finally, we apply the adjustments discussed in Chapter Three to estimate the benefits of all four disease management programs combined, after aligning the MEPS expenditures with those in the national Health Expenditures (NHE) and projecting utilization, expenditures, and outcomes to future years.

Program Design

Currently, there are two approaches to disease management. In the more common approach, a payer organization contracts with a disease management company or forms an internal disease-management unit. On paper, the programs operated by these disease managers include all the DMAA components in one form or another.

But because the disease manager works outside the normal process of care—trying to affect care indirectly through communications with patients and providers—these programs often fall short of the DMAA ideal. The care process really does not change. In the second approach, a provider—often a primary care physician—will create his or her own disease management program. Because he or she is more closely involved in the care process, we feel that this approach has the greater promise, and it is the one we have analyzed.

It is not easy for a physician to establish a chronic disease management program. But starting in approximately 1998, Dr. Ed Wagner developed the Chronic Care Model[2] (Bodenheimer, Wagner, and Grumbach, 2002a, b), a template for provider-based chronic disease management. In 2000, the Institute for Healthcare Improvement (IHI)[3] made this model the basis for several of its "breakthrough collaboratives," a model that IHI developed to help healthcare organizations make breakthroughs in quality improvements while reducing costs.

Most disease-management and chronic-care programs reported in the literature possess similar elements. We exploited the similarities to define a generic care program having the following components:

- Identify a patient with the target condition, enroll him or her, and perform an initial assessment. The initial assessment involves a care team consisting of a primary care physician (PCP) and/or a specialist, a nurse, and the patient. The PCP or specialist performs the necessary diagnostic tests and evaluations. The nurse evaluates the lifestyle of the patient for factors that may contribute to the disease or its effects, and assesses the patient's knowledge and readiness for change. Starting from evidence-based guidelines, the team begins to formulate a care plan tailored to this patient's particular circumstances.
- Provide the patient with initial education and training. This component is usually delivered in a group, although it can be done one on one, either face to face or by phone, through video and printed media, or over the Internet. Generally, this component is delivered by a nurse, nurse-educator, social worker, or pharmacist. A basic element of every disease management program, it is often used in the literature reviews to distinguish disease management programs from regular care.
- Provide the patient with individualized, ongoing education, monitoring, and feedback. This component includes compliance assessment, monitoring of the changes in the symptoms of the disease, and ongoing individual or targeted

---

[2] See http://www.improvingchroniccare.org for more information on the Chronic Care Model.

[3] See http://www.ihi.org.

education. It can be delivered during home visits by a nurse or through tele-communication channels.

- Provide reminders to patients of scheduled visits, tests, educational sessions, etc. A nurse or clerical worker may coordinate this component.
- Perform ongoing evaluation and treatment (care plan) adjustment. This component includes all regular tests and evaluations, and follows the frequency stated in guidelines. It occurs mostly during regular visits to the physician's office, and it requires time from both PCP and nurse. When appropriate, it includes regular visits to a specialist (e.g., diabetics require regular retinal examinations by an ophthalmologist).
- Other activities depend on the specifics of the disease (e.g., group therapy).

These are only the direct components. The DMAA definition also calls for measurement, evaluation, and reporting of outcomes. There will also be the usual management (e.g., hiring and scheduling of staff) and administrative (e.g., billing) activities.

HIT in Disease Management

Information systems play many roles in disease management. All disease management programs identify patients by scanning an electronic file to determine who has the target condition. Payer-based disease-management programs often scan a claims file. Provider-based systems scan an Electronic Medical Record (EMR). Once patients are enrolled, data from this file populate a patient registry, which is used for tracking the events that make up the disease management program.

The patient registry—which may be a stand-alone HIT application or a feature of an EMR—incorporates the evidence-based practice guidelines referred to in the DMAA definition above. These guidelines serve as a template for a plan of care for each enrolled patient. As data are entered into the registry, it can automatically compare the actual care to the plan and notify both provider and patient of discrepancies. For the most part, such notices will be reminders that an event is due.

Initial patient education is probably best accomplished face to face, but much ongoing education, monitoring, and feedback can be handled electronically. For example, Health Hero Network[4] provides a device (the Health Buddy, a two-way communication device) that supports disease management of patients with chronic conditions. Each day, a short questionnaire is downloaded to the Health Buddy, asking the patient about symptoms and probing the patient's knowledge about his or her medications and dietary restrictions. The completed questionnaire is fed back to the provider, who can then revise the patient's treatment regime (e.g., adjust medica-

---

[4] See http://www.healthhero.com; last accessed July 2005.

tions) in a timely fashion, and can address any weak areas in the patient's knowledge and understanding.

The disease management programs we envision require a good deal of self-care by patients. Self-care is a major departure from the traditional paradigm of medicine, in which healthcare is a commodity delivered by providers to largely passive patients. Of course, even in a traditional medical practice, the doctor must rely on the patient to fill the prescription and take the pills—something that patients do only about half the time (Roter et al., 1998; Haynes, McDonald, and Garg, 2002). Disease management depends for its success on patients becoming their own health care providers, not just in the days after a surgery or a bout of fever, but for a lifetime. In Chapter Eight, we discuss what proportion of patients we think might be taught, cajoled, or browbeaten to accept this role, and how can HIT help.

Estimating the Costs of Disease Management Programs

We estimated the cost per managed patient per year based on labor resources spent directly on the components listed above. We used literature, medical expertise, and common sense to assess how much labor input each instance of a component requires, and how many instances of that component would be performed per patient per year. Both the number of instances and the labor per instance should vary with the severity of the disease. Thus, for each disease, we separated the patient population into several medically relevant risk groups. Similarly, there should be more activity in the first year a patient is enrolled, and less in subsequent years. For example, general education might be needed only at the beginning of the program. Finally, the level of Health Information Technology (HIT) employed could make a difference in the cost. Thus, we built two scenarios: (1) basic HIT, including an Electronic Medical Record System (EMR-S) with a disease registry; and (2) advanced HIT, with special disease management functions, such as automatic outreach, automated phone or Web-based education and monitoring, and disease management–related decision support. For each disease, then, we estimated annual per-patient costs for two HIT scenarios times two years (first and subsequent), times the number of risk groups for that disease.

We illustrate our method using diabetes management as the example. From our consultations with a physician and a review of medical literature, we defined two risk groups in the diabetes population. The high-risk group consists of Type I (insulin-dependent) diabetics, plus Type II diabetics who have developed complications, have excessively high HbA1c[5] levels, or have comorbidities that put them at higher risk. In

---

[5] HbA1c, or glycosylated hemoglobin, is a measure of average blood-sugar levels over the past three months. Normally, the HbA1c form of hemoglobin is only 3–6.5 percent of total hemoglobin. In diabetics whose blood sugar is not under good control, it can be much higher. The goal for diabetics is to keep blood sugar controlled, as indicated by an HbA1c measurement of 7 percent or less.

total, about 30 percent of diabetics are in this high-risk group. This proportion agrees with the disease management literature, which puts about 30 percent of diabetic patients in the category with greater care needs (Domurat, 1999).

Table 6.1 shows our labor estimates for a diabetic patient in the high-risk group in her first year of the program. Each panel of the table presents data for a different component of the program, and each row within a panel contains data for a different type of labor.

The diabetes management model we developed starts with an assessment of the patient by a medical doctor, specialist, and/or nurse, which we assumed would last up to an hour in total. In the subsequent years, assessment is a part of an annual planned visit to the doctor, and its duration is reduced.

Education and training on self-management is a cornerstone of every diabetes management program. Most of the comprehensive diabetes care programs offer group education sessions for six to 18 patients, which last about 1.5 to 2 hours and are held two to eight times, mostly in the first year of the program (e.g., Sadur et al., 1999; Wagner et al., 2001; Sidorov et al., 2000). For the most part nurse-educators, nurses, or pharmacists conduct these group sessions, but occasionally they involve specialists (diabetologists, nutritionists, etc.). Alternative programs deliver individualized education during a visit or through phone calls by a nurse, and mostly target patients from the high-risk group (e.g., Aubert et al., 1998; Piette et al., 2001). We assumed that the education program includes about five group education and training sessions for about seven high-risk or 12 low-risk patients in the first year of the program and one per year in all subsequent years.

Monitoring, feedback, and targeted education become more important for more-severe diabetes cases. This component involves reporting symptoms, behavioral changes, and glucose levels to the nurse and getting her feedback and advice. The literature mentions biweekly to quarterly monitoring, depending on the severity of the case. We assumed a bimonthly checkup by a nurse for the low-risk group, and a checkup 10 times per year for the high-risk group. Monitoring is reduced in the subsequent years of the program, as the patient learns self-monitoring, to quarterly and eight times per year, respectively. In addition, the physician devotes his or her time to these monitoring activities during the annual checkup or quarterly visits.

We assumed the duration to be about 12 minutes, on average, for the low-risk case and 20 minutes for the high-risk case.

According to guidelines, a diabetes patient should have his HbA1c tested every six months and his or her feet examined every three months. Thus, we assumed four visits per year, with a nurse spending about 15–20 minutes per visit and a doctor spending from 10 to 20 minutes on further evaluations and treatment adjustments, depending on the severity of the case.

Table 6.1
Labor Estimates for a High-Risk Diabetic Patient in Year 1 of the Program

Program Component	Times per Year	Duration (hr)	Percent of Patients	Number of Patients per Instance	"Face" Time per Patient (hr)	Prep Time (hr)	Total Provider Time per Patient (hr)
Assessment and development of a treatment plan							
Physician	1	0.5	100%	1	0.5		0.5
Specialist (diabetologist)	1	0.5	100%	1	0.5		0.5
General education about diabetes (in a group)							
Nurse	4	2	50%	7	0.57	0.8	1.37
Specialist (e.g., pharmacist, nutritionist, diabetologist)	1	2	100%	7	0.29	0.2	0.49
Individualized-education, monitoring, and feedback							
Nurse	10	0.3	100%	1	3	1	4
Physician	1	0.3	100%	1	0.3	0.1	0.4
Ongoing evaluation and treatment							
Nurse	4	0.25	100%	1	1		1
Physician	4	0.25	100%	1	1		1
Specialist Care							
Ophthalmologist	1	0.25	100%	1	0.25		0.25
Specialist (e.g., podiatrist, endocrinologist)	1	0.35	100%	1	0.35	0.1	0.45
Group therapy							
Nurse	1	1	70%	10	0.07	0.1	0.17
Outreach (telephone reminders)							
Nurse	10	0.1	90%	1	0.9		0.9

Diabetes guidelines also call for an annual checkup by an ophthalmologist. Some programs deliver this service in one of the group education sessions. We assumed that the entire group gets eye exams at the same time, which take about 15 to 20 minutes per patient. Referrals to other specialists are a part of regular chronic care. We assumed that 30 percent of the low-risk population and 100 percent of the high-risk population need a retinal exam once a year.

Outreach reminds patients of their upcoming appointments for tests, group education sessions, etc., and could be merged with phone-based monitoring. We assumed that each telephone call takes about 5 minutes and happens from five to 10 times per year, depending on the severity of the disease.

A group therapy session to exchange experiences among diabetic patients is also deemed beneficial in many disease management programs, but it does not require 100-percent attendance. We assumed that 70 percent of high-risk patients (50 percent of low-risk patients) would attend in the first year of the program. Attendance drops to 30 percent for both risk groups in the subsequent years.

From these data, we calculated the hours a provider spends face to face with a patient in each activity, on a per-patient basis (column 6). We added "preparation time" (column 7) to obtain "total provider time per patient" (column 8).

We estimated three kinds of labor: a doctor's time costs $60 per hour, on average; a nurse's time costs $23 per hour; and any other labor costs $20 per hour.[6] We estimated benefits to be 30 percent of wages.[7] We did not explicitly account for the extra costs of start-up, nor did we explicitly consider the resources used for indirect or support activities. Instead, we added an overhead cost equal to 80 percent of direct labor costs. Physician practices appear to have overhead factors (as defined here) of around 60 percent (AMA, 2003), and we have boosted the figure a bit to allow for amortization of program start-up costs.

In Table 6.1, all providers are either doctors or nurses. Summing over all activities, we found that each patient consumes 3.59 physician hours and 7.44 nurse hours during the year. At the prices mentioned, these hours have a total cost of $811.22, counting direct salaries plus benefits plus overhead.

For low-risk patients, the total provider time per patient is 5 hours by a nurse and 2.5 hours by a doctor in the first year, and 2 hours by a doctor and 3 hours by a nurse in subsequent years. Sidorov et al. (2002) report on a program that employed 51 disease management nurses for over 4,000 patients. If there are 230 8-hour workdays per year, the nurses spent over 20 hours per patient, which exceeds our estimate several times. If these data are from a newly implemented program, they will include some start-up training time for nurses. In addition, some nurse time may be spent on overhead functions and some on research-related activities, such as information collection.

Estimating the Benefits of Disease Management

We estimated most benefits by combining the trajectory file we assembled from the MEPS (see Chapter Two) with factors obtained from the literature. As an example, Table 6.2 summarizes the data in the trajectory file for the 11.5 million people

---

[6] Bureau of Labor Statistics, http://www.bls.gov/oes/oes_dl.htm; last accessed July 2005.

[7] Bureau of Labor Statistics, http://www.bls.gov/ncs/ect/home.htm; last accessed July 2005.

Table 6.2
Summary of Data for Diabetics from the Trajectory File

	Diabetics				
	Events with Diabetes Diagnosis	Other Events	Total	Comparison Group	Difference
Utilization Measures (millions)					
Inpatient Stays	0.6	3.7	4.3	1.9	−2.5
Inpatient Nights	4.4	28.5	32.9	12.2	−20.7
Hospital Ambulatory Visits	3.6	16.7	20.3	11.1	−9.3
Office Visits, MD	32.9	57.3	90.3	51.2	−39.1
Office Visits, Non-MD	5.3	20.3	25.6	18.3	−7.4
Expenditures ($billions)					
Hospital	$5.4	$35.7	$41.1	$18.6	−$22.5
Physician	$3.8	$12.6	$16.4	$9.3	−$7.1
Rx	$5.9	$12.3	$18.1	$6.5	−$11.6
Other	$0.5	$12.9	$13.5	$8.4	−$5.1
Total	$15.6	$73.5	$89.1	$42.8	−$46.3
Days Affected (millions)					
Schooldays Lost			1.0	0.5	−0.5
Workdays Lost			35.1	26.1	−8.9
Days Sick Abed			188.8	77.7	−111.1
Mortality (thousands)					
Deaths			345.0	232.5	−112.5

diagnosed with diabetes. The top panel of the table gives utilization data, the second panel gives expenditure data, and the remaining two panels provide health outcomes data. The first three columns give data on diabetics, the fourth column gives data on a comparison group of 11.5 million people who do not have diabetes, and the final column gives the difference between the comparison group and the "Total" column for diabetics. We selected the comparison group to have the same distribution over age, gender, and ethnicity as the population of diabetics.

The first column for diabetics contains data on events that carry a diabetes diagnosis (hospital stays, visits to the emergency room or hospital outpatient department, office visits to physicians and other providers, prescription drugs). The second column contains data for events that do not carry a diabetes diagnosis. Health outcomes cannot be attributed to diagnoses using the data in the MEPS, so we placed them in the "Total" column.

To model short-term effects of a diabetes management program, we altered selected elements that contribute to columns 1 and 2. For a typical disease management program, doing so mostly means reducing emergency room (ER) visits and hospital stays, increasing office visits to physicians, and adding dollars for outreach activities, such as nursing advice lines. One might think that the effects of a disease management program would be confined to column 1, but the literature suggests that this is not so. For diabetes, about half of all ER visits and hospital stays are eliminated by disease management, not just visits and stays for diabetes.

We assumed that other than ER visits, most ambulatory care associated with the target condition—we assumed 90 percent—will be replaced by the activities of our comprehensive disease management program, including both office visits and visits to hospital outpatient departments. To derive the net benefit of the disease management, therefore, we replaced 90 percent of the current unplanned provider visits with the disease management program's planned provider visits, telemonitoring and phone-based support, etc.

Disease management can also improve on such outcomes as workdays and schooldays lost, as well as on additional days spent in bed. As mentioned earlier, the trajectory file provides these quantities for each respondent, but it does not attribute them to medical conditions. When the literature provided a percentage reduction in these measures, we applied that reduction to the MEPS quantities. Even when the literature provided no guide, we compared the MEPS quantities for people with the target condition to the same quantities for a demographically matched comparison group of people without the condition, as a rough guide to the social benefits of disease management.

Spreadsheets

We built our disease management cost models as Excel files. To estimate benefits, we extracted data from the MEPS files on people with each of the conditions we examined and imported those data into Excel files for analysis. All eight Excel files are available at http://www.rand.org/publications/MG/MG408 and on the compact disc (CD) included with printed copies of this monograph. The file names are as follows:

- Diabetes management costs.xls
- Diabetes management effects.xls
- CHF management costs.xls
- CHF management effects.xls
- Asthma management costs.xls
- Asthma management effects.xls
- COPD management costs.xls
- COPD management effects.xls.

We now turn to our analysis of each of the four conditions.

Diabetes Management

The Population with Diabetes

We take a respondent in the trajectory file to have diabetes if the Clinical Condition Codes (AHRQ CCC) and 3-digit *International Classification of Diseases,* Revision 9 (ICD-9) codes (CDC ICD-9) in Table 6.3 are associated with that respondent.

We discovered that it is unwise to use CCC=050 for identifying diabetes with complications. Instead, we have identified other diagnoses considered to be complications of diabetes, as shown in Table 6.4.

According to the MEPS data, 11.5 million people in the United States have been diagnosed with diabetes. This number agrees well with an estimate by the National Institute of Diabetes and Digestive and Kidney Diseases (NIDDK).[8] NIDDK's website indicates that approximately 18.2 million people in the United States have diabetes, and 13 million of them have been diagnosed.

Table 6.3
MEPS Diagnoses Included in Diabetes

CCC	CCC Label	ICD9.3	ICD9.3 Label
049	Diabetes mellitus without complications	250	DIABETES MELLITUS*
		790	ABNORMAL BLOOD FINDINGS*
		791	ABNORMAL URINE FINDINGS*
050	Diabetes mellitus with complications	250	DIABETES MELLITUS*

NOTE: The asterisk is part of the ICD9.3 label. It does not refer to this note.

_____

[8] See http://www.diabetes.niddk.nih.gov/dm/pubs/overview/index.htm; accessed January 1, 2005.

Table 6.4
MEPS Diagnoses Identified as Complications of Diabetes

CCC	CCC Label	ICD9.3	ICD9.3 Label
		Chronic Renal Failure	
158	Chronic renal failure	585	CHRONIC RENAL FAILURE
		792	ABN FIND-OTH BODY SUBST*
		V42	ORGAN TRANSPLANT STATUS*
		V45	OTH POSTSURGICAL STATES*
		V56	DIALYSIS ENCOUNTER*
		Lower Limb Involvement	
114	Peripheral and visceral atherosclerosis	440	ATHEROSCLEROSIS*
199	Chronic ulcer of skin	707	CHRONIC ULCER OF SKIN*
211	Other connective tissue disease	V49	LIMB PROBLEM/PROBLEM NEC*
		Retinopathy	
087	Retinal detachments, defects, vascular occlusion, and retinopathy	362	RETINAL DISORDERS NEC*
		Neuropathy	
095	Other nervous system disorders	337	AUTONOMIC NERVE DISORDER*
		355	MONONEURITIS LEG*
		Hypertension	
098	Essential hypertension	401	ESSENTIAL HYPERTENSION*
099	Hypertension with complications and secondary hypertension	401	ESSENTIAL HYPERTENSION*
		402	HYPERTENSIVE HEART DIS*
		403	HYPERTENSIVE RENAL DIS*
		459	OTH CIRCULATORY DISEASE*
		Hyperlipidemia	
053	Disorders of lipid metabolism	272	DIS OF LIPOID METABOLISM*
		Coronary Artery Disease	
100	Acute myocardial infarction	410	ACUTE MYOCARDIAL INFARCT*
101	Coronary atherosclerosis and other heart disease	411	OTH AC ISCHEMIC HRT DIS*
		412	OLD MYOCARDIAL INFARCT
		413	ANGINA PECTORIS*
		414	OTH CHR ISCHEMIC HRT DIS*
		V45	OTH POSTSURGICAL STATES*

Table 6.4—Continued

CCC	CCC Label	ICD9.3	ICD9.3 Label
	Cerebrovascular Disease/Stroke		
109	Acute cerebrovascular disease	430	SUBARACHNOID HEMORRHAGE
		431	INTRACEREBRAL HEMORRHAGE
		432	INTRACRANIAL HEM NEC/NOS*
		434	CEREBRAL ARTERY OCCLUS*
		436	CVA
		437	OTH CEREBROVASC DISEASE*
110	Occlusion or stenosis of precerebral arteries	433	PRECEREBRAL OCCLUSION*
112	Transient cerebral ischemia	435	TRANSIENT CEREB ISCHEMIA*
113	Late effects of cerebrovascular disease	438	LATE EFF CEREBROVASC DIS*
	Heart Failure		
108	Congestive heart failure, nonhypertensive	428	HEART FAILURE*
	Other Heart Diseases		
096	Heart valve disorders	394	DISEASES OF MITRAL VALVE*
		397	ENDOCARDIAL DISEASE NEC*
		424	OTH ENDOCARDIAL DISEASE*
		785	CARDIOVASCULAR SYS SYMP*
		V42	ORGAN TRANSPLANT STATUS*
		V43	ORGAN REPLACEMENT NEC*
097	Peri-, endo-, and myocarditis, cardiomyopathy (except that caused by tuberculosis or sexually transmitted disease)	139	LATE EFFECT INFECT NEC*
		391	RHEUM FEV W HEART INVOLV*
		398	OTH RHEUMATIC HEART DIS*
		420	ACUTE PERICARDITIS*
		422	ACUTE MYOCARDITIS*
		423	OTH PERICARDIAL DISEASE*
		425	CARDIOMYOPATHY*
		429	ILL-DEFINED HEART DIS*
102	Nonspecific chest pain	786	RESP SYS/OTH CHEST SYMP*
103	Pulmonary heart disease	415	ACUTE PULMONARY HRT DIS*
		416	CHR PULMONARY HEART DIS*
104	Other and ill-defined heart disease	414	OTH CHR ISCHEMIC HRT DIS*
105	Conduction disorders	426	CONDUCTION DISORDERS*
		V45	OTH POSTSURGICAL STATES*
		V53	ADJUSTMENT OF OTH DEVICE*

Table 6.4—Continued

CCC	CCC Label	ICD9.3	ICD9.3 Label
		Other Heart Diseases—Continued	
106	Cardiac dysrhythmias	427	CARDIAC DYSRHYTHMIAS*
		785	CARDIOVASCULAR SYS SYMP*
107	Cardiac arrest and ventricular fibrillation	427	CARDIAC DYSRHYTHMIAS*

NOTE: The asterisk is part of the ICD9.3 label. It does not refer to this note.
NEC = Not Elsewhere Considered.
NOS = Not Otherwise Specified.

Diabetes Management Costs

Table 6.5 shows the costs per patient for all the different diabetes scenarios. The discussion above explains why costs are higher in the first year than in subsequent years, and why low-risk patients are less costly than high-risk patients. But how does a high level of automation (advanced HIT in place of basic HIT) reduce costs?

Advanced HIT would replace general education provided in a group with self-education through a computer program, which does not require the provider to spend time. A couple of nurse-led group classes would be provided to a segment of the population (50 percent) to train and augment the computer-based education. In addition, e-forums would replace group support sessions. Phone-based outreach by a nurse would be replaced by an automated email or automated telephone calls. Monitoring could be partially automated by Health Buddy–like devices, which allow tele-monitoring through the Internet or a touch-tone phone. However, a nurse would need to follow up on any red flags generated by telemonitoring. We reduced time spent on these functions by 50 percent. Similarly, we reduced time spent on assessment by 50 percent, assuming that HIT would speed up the process of pulling together all relevant data, providing decision support, generating a treatment plan, and developing a disease-management plan based on a computer-based questionnaire of the patient's behavioral factors, symptoms, readiness for change, knowledge, etc.

Table 6.5
Cost of Diabetes Management per Patient per Year

HIT Level	Risk Group	First Year	Subsequent Years
Basic	Low	$570.64	$344.27
Basic	High	$811.22	$652.52
Advanced	Low	$275.31	$227.85
Advanced	High	$478.54	$433.86

For simplicity, we computed an average cost per patient for diabetes disease management. We weighted the costs of the first and subsequent years by the ratio of diabetes incidence to prevalence, which we estimated to be about 10 percent.[9] From the MEPS data, 7.2 million diabetics—approximately 63 percent of the total number of diabetics—have no complications other than possibly hypertension or hyperlipidemia. Thus, we put 63 percent of the population in the low-risk group and the remaining 37 percent in the high-risk group.[10] The average costs become $478.46 per patient per year for basic HIT versus $308.72 per patient per year for advanced HIT.

To check this figure, consider the following: The MEPS file shows almost 33 million office visits to physicians that are associated with a diagnosis of diabetes. The total expenditure on these visits is $3.16 billion, for an expenditure of $96 per visit. According to Table 6.1, the diabetes management program requires the patient to make four visits per year to his or her physician for ongoing evaluation and treatment, and we suppose that the other in-office services can be performed during these visits. Thus, the per-visit cost of our diabetes management program is very similar to the cost of current diabetes-related office visits.

Diabetes Management Benefits

Next, we describe how we estimated the short-term benefits of diabetes management. As Bodenheimer, Wagner, and Grumbach (2002b) remark,

> In contrast with programs for CHF and asthma, which may produce cost savings almost immediately through reduced hospital and ED use, programs that improve diabetic glycemic control would be expected to show savings only throughout the long term, with reduced vascular complications. Surprisingly, some studies have shown that improved diabetic care can save money in the short run.

Table 6.6 presents our estimates of the short-term effects of our model diabetes management program on healthcare utilization, healthcare expenditures, and selected outcomes. We estimated these quantities by generating a table such as Table 6.2 from the MEPS database and applying factors from the published literature. We obtained three values for most factors: low, middle, and high. We used the middle values to estimate the quantities in the first three columns. The last two columns

---

[9] The ratio of new cases diagnosed in 2002 (1.3 million) to the diabetic population (13 million) is about 10 percent, based on current Centers for Disease Control and Prevention (CDC) data (http://www.cdc.gov/diabetes/statistics/prev/national/figpersons.htm; last accessed August 3, 2005). However, other resources, such as Norris et al. (2002), provide alternative data that give the ratio as about 5 percent (0.79 million divided by 16 million).

[10] A targeted program might preferentially enroll high-risk diabetics. This is a common practice.

Table 6.6
Effect of Diabetes Management on Utilization, Expenditures, and Outcomes[a]

	Under 65	65 and Older	Total	Range of Total Low	Range of Total High
Population (millions)	6.2	5.3	11.5		
Utilization Measures (millions)					
Inpatient Stays	−0.9	−1.3	−2.2	−1.1	−3.3
Inpatient Nights	−5.9	−10.6	−16.4	−8.2	−24.7
Hosp Outpatient + ER Visits	−1.8	−1.1	−2.9	−1.9	−3.8
Office Visits	−15.2	−14.4	−29.6	−28.0	−31.3
Disease Mgt Visits	24.8	21.3	46.0		
Expenditures ($billions)					
Hospital	−$7.4	−$11.1	−$18.5	−$9.5	−$27.4
Physician	−$2.5	−$3.0	−$5.4	−$4.0	−$6.8
Program Cost	$3.0	$2.5	$5.5	$5.5	$5.5
Rx	$0.0	$0.0	$0.0	$1.2	−$1.2
Total	−$6.8	−$11.5	−$18.4	−$6.8	−$29.9
Days Affected (millions)					
Schooldays Lost	−0.5	0.0	−0.5		
Workdays Lost	−8.1	−0.8	−8.9		
Total Days Abed	−59.7	−51.4	−111.1		
Mortality (thousands)					
Deaths	−51.9	−60.7	−112.5		

[a]Deaths in the "Under 65" column were estimated from 36 observations from the MEPS dataset, and deaths in the "65 and Older" column from 111 observations. All other items were estimated from more than 2,000 observations. The Agency for Healthcare Research and Quality (AHRQ) declines to report estimates made from fewer than 100 observations.

show the range of the "Total" column, calculated using the low and high values for the factors. We make no adjustments for MEPS respondents who might already have been in diabetes management programs, which results in an overestimate of both benefits and costs.

Effects on Utilization Measures. Factors for estimating the short-term benefits of diabetes management come from literature that evaluates the outcomes of relatively comprehensive programs one to two years after the beginning of the programs. On the high end, Sadur et al. (1999) claim about an 82-percent reduction in all-cause hospitalizations in the intervention group as compared with controls, whereas Wagner et al. (2001) and Sidorov et al. (2002) report about a 40-percent reduction in inpatient days. Other disease management programs—Steffens (2000), Villagra and Ahmed (2004), Bott et al. (2000), Rubin, Dietrich, and Hawk (1998)—achieved reductions in hospitalizations or hospital days in the range of 20 to 30 percent. From this literature, we estimated an assumed reduction in hospital stays and expenditures of 50 percent (average), 25 percent (lower bound), and 75 percent (upper bound). Emergency room visits are also well studied in the literature. Leiberman (2001) and Wagner et al. (2001) claim a reduction of 77 percent and 95 percent, whereas Sidorov et al. (2002) and Villagra and Ahmed (2004) report reductions of 13 percent and 23 percent, respectively. For our model, we assumed the same reduction rates for emergency room visits as for inpatient stays: 25, 50, and 75 percent.

We supposed that disease management eliminates the majority of unscheduled acute care, including ambulatory care, and replaces it with planned care. Thus, we assumed that the disease management program would eliminate 90 percent of hospital outpatient department or office visits to physicians that are associated with a diabetes diagnosis. But the disease management program itself requires office visits to a physician, so we added four visits per year for each enrollee. There is very sparse evidence that can help us evaluate the effect of disease management on ambulatory visits. However, our assumption is roughly consistent with the results from Sadur et al. (1999), who claim that net visits to physicians were reduced by 17 percent and that visits to nonphysicians increased 8 times as a result of a disease management program.

Effects on Expenditures. We reduced expenditures on each event type by the same percentage as we reduced those on utilization. We then summarized expenditure reductions by recipient. Hospitals receive part of the expenditures from ER visits, inpatient stays, and outpatient visits, and physicians bill separately for the rest. Physicians bear the entire reduction in expenditures on office visits.

We have calculated the program cost at $478.46 per enrollee per year, assuming that all people diagnosed with diabetes are enrolled. As mentioned earlier, this is the average cost per person for basic HIT. We have reported this number separately, although we suspect most of it would be paid to physician practices.

The literature is inconsistent about the theoretical and empirical effect of diabetes management on drug utilization. Studies usually mention that, in the short term, drug use would increase as the patients improve compliance with their drug regime as a result of disease management efforts; however, in the long run, the need for more drugs would be eliminated when disease management successfully prevents the exacerbation of the condition. Very few empirical studies have formally evaluated this hypothesis: Villagra and Ahmed (2004) claim an 8-percent reduction in drug costs, whereas Berger et al. (2001) predict a 5-percent increase. Without better empirical evidence, we assumed the effect on the drug costs to range from –20 to +20 percent, with 0-percent average change.

Effects on Outcomes. We also estimated the effect of our diabetes management program on days spent sick in bed, days lost from school, and days lost from work. Our method was to compare two populations from the MEPS. One is the population diagnosed with diabetes. The other is a comparison group with the same distribution over sex, age categories, and ethnicities. The numbers in Table 6.6 are the differences between the two groups, and they represent reductions of 59 percent in days spent sick in bed, 53 percent in schooldays lost, and 25 percent in workdays lost. These, of course, are only selected outcomes; they do not account for all differences between the two populations.

There was very limited information in the literature to which we could compare these estimates. Wagner et al. (2001) report a 40-percent reduction in days spent in bed, whereas Bott et al. (2000) report a 60-percent reduction in missed workdays.

It is common to find estimates of the cost of a disease to the nation as a whole. These estimates include direct costs for health care, plus such indirect costs as lost productivity and the value of years of life lost. By assigning costs to days sick in bed and to days of work or school lost, we can get a sense of the effect of disease management on these indirect costs. Suppose we value avoiding a day sick in bed at $50,[11] a schoolday at $20,[12] and a workday at $140.[13] Then our comprehensive diabetes management program, applied to all 11.5 million diabetics, would produce $6.81 billion in indirect savings from the reductions in sick days shown in Table 6.6.

We have not estimated the short-term effect of diabetes management on mortality, but here are some facts from which we can develop a very rough sense of the possibilities. The National Center for Health Statistics reports 69,301 deaths from diabetes mellitus in 2000 (NCHS GMWK, n.d.). These are counts of death certificates that gave "diabetes mellitus" as the cause of death; they do not include deaths for which diabetes was considered only a contributory factor.

The MEPS shows 345,000 deaths from all causes among people with diabetes—about 3 percent of diabetics per year. A comparison group without diabetes, but matched on age, sex, and ethnicity, shows 233,000 deaths, for a difference of 112,000. This figure might be closer than the CDC figure to the number of deaths that might be postponed by better management of diabetes.

We estimated from the literature that diabetes management cuts hospitalizations by half. Assuming that most deaths of diabetics occur in a hospital, we took half of the above figures to be a rough estimate of deaths postponed—i.e., 35,000 to 57,000.

---

[11] This is the California minimum wage ($6.26/hour) for 8 hours.

[12] This is approximately the amount a California school district receives from the state per pupil-day of attendance.

[13] This is close to the average salary for all occupations, as reported by the Bureau of Labor Statistics.

CHF Management

The Population with CHF

We took a respondent in the trajectory file to have CHF if the pair of a CCC and a 3-digit ICD-9 code in Table 6.7 was associated with that respondent.

As a condition, CHF is somewhat ambiguous. From the MEPS, we calculated that 1.42 million people have the condition as we define it. Yet there are many papers that claim a much higher prevalence—for example, "nearly 5 million," according to Jessup and Brozena (2003). Similarly, Gillespie (2001) reports that 4 million people have been diagnosed with CHF. On the other hand, Brown (2000) claims that "over two million people in the United States are affected by this syndrome . . ." (in Kerr et al., eds., 2000, p. 179).

The difference lies, no doubt, in just what diagnoses are included in CHF. For example, Brown includes the 5-digit ICD-9 codes in Table 6.8. The MEPS reports only the first three digits of the ICD-9 code, but it shows about 6 million people with a CCC=104 (Other and ill-defined heart disease) paired with ICD9.3=429 (ILL-DEFINED HEART DIS*).

CHF Management Costs

To construct our model of CHF management costs, we consulted the National Pharmaceutical Council (NPC) report (NPC, 2004c), which reviews over 50 programs, plus articles that describe particular comprehensive programs in further detail. The review by Gillespie (2001) describes a number of CHF disease management programs and their common features, as well as their achieved savings and benefits. The other sources that we used to derive the numbers for our model of CHF disease management include Vaccaro et al. (2001), Eliaszadeh et al. (2001), Clarke and Nash (2002), Knox and Mischke (1999), West et al. (1997), Shah et al. (1998), Cline et al. (1998), and Rich et al. (1995).

The severity of CHF cases is well reflected in the New York Heart Association (NYHA) classification. With the help of a clinician, we constructed three risk groups with different disease management programs: NYHA classes 1 and 2 (approximately

Table 6.7
MEPS Diagnoses Included in CHF

CCC	CCC Label	ICD9.3	ICD9.3 Label
108	Congestive heart failure, nonhypertensive	428	HEART FAILURE*

NOTE: The asterisk is part of the ICD9.3 label. It does not refer to this note.

Table 6.8
Definition of CHF According to Kerr et al., eds. (2000)

ICD-9	ICD-9 Label
428.xx	HEART FAILURE*
398.91	RHEUMATIC HEART FAILURE
402.01	MAL HYPERT HRT DIS W CHF
402.11	BENIGN HYP HRT DIS W CHF
402.91	HYPERTEN HEART DIS W CHF
404.01	MAL HYPER HRT/REN W CHF OCT89—
404.03	MAL HYP HRT/REN W CHF&RF OCT89—
404.11	BEN HYPER HRT/REN W CHF OCT89—
404.13	BEN HYP HRT/REN W CHF&RF OCT89—
404.91	HYPER HRT/REN NOS W CHF OCT89—
404.93	HYP HT/REN NOS W CHF&RF OCT89—
425.4	PRIM CARDIOMYOPATHY NEC
429.1	MYOCARDIAL DEGENERATION

NOTE: The asterisk is part of the ICD-9 label. It does not refer to this note.
NEC = not elsewhere considered.

55 percent of patients); class 3 (about 30 percent); and class 4 (about 15 percent). Most CHF management programs are directed toward class 3 and 4 patients. Table 6.9 shows our estimated costs of managing such patients.

According to Gillespie (2001), there are 400,000 new cases each year, resulting in a ratio of incidence to prevalence of 10 percent. This suggests that if we enrolled people in a CHF management program when they were first diagnosed, 10 percent of them would be in their first year. However, they are typically not enrolled until their cases become more severe (NYHA classes 3 and 4). About half of the people in classes 3 and 4 die each year (Jessup and Brozena, 2003), so we weight the first- and

Table 6.9
Cost of CHF Management per Patient per Year

HIT Level	Severity	First Year	Subsequent Years
Basic	Classes 1&2	$413.37	$228.06
Basic	Class 3	$818.27	$460.95
Basic	Class 4	$1,298.85	$717.78
Advanced	Classes 1&2	$253.73	$203.91
Advanced	Class 3	$596.09	$422.94
Advanced	Class 4	$786.87	$422.94

subsequent-year costs equally. (Clarke and Nash [2002] report much lower mortality rates—6 percent in the first year for people enrolled in their program—so perhaps we should weight subsequent years more heavily.) We assumed that class 3 and class 4 patients are enrolled in proportion to their relative numbers (twice as many class 3 patients), but we only enroll a few classes 1 and 2 patients. We weight classes 1 and 2 costs by 10 percent, class 3 by 60 percent, and class 4 by 30 percent. The average costs become $718.33 per patient per year for basic HIT and $510.36 per patient per year for advanced HIT.

CHF Management Benefits

Table 6.10 presents our estimates of the effects of our model CHF management program on healthcare utilization, healthcare expenditures, and selected outcomes. We estimated these quantities by generating a table such as Table 6.2 from the MEPS database and applying factors from the published literature. We obtained three values for most factors: low, middle, and high. We used the middle values to estimate the quantities in the first three columns. The last two columns show the range of the "Total" column, calculated using the low and high values for the factors. We make no adjustments for MEPS respondents who might already have been in CHF management programs, which results in an overestimate of both benefits and costs.

Effects on Utilization Measures. Philbin et al. (2000) produced a systematic review of comprehensive CHF management programs. According to this review, six studies reported a 50- to 85-percent reduction in hospitalizations, and one study reported a 36-percent reduction. Newer sources also demonstrate a substantial decrease in hospitalizations: around 50 percent by Vaccaro et al. (2001) and Eliaszadeh et al. (2001), and 22 percent by Clarke and Nash (2002). These sources also provide the results on the reductions in ER visits: 73, 52, and 25 percent, correspondingly. West et al. (1997) reports around a 73-percent reduction in CHF-related ER visits, and Gillespie (2001) reports a 67-percent reduction in CHF-related ER visits and a 53-percent reduction in all-cause ER visits. Given this information, we assumed 30-percent (lower bound), 50-percent (middle case), and 75-percent (higher bound) reductions in both hospital stays and ER visits for all causes.

According to West et al. (1997), the net effect of the CHF management was a 31-percent reduction in visits to cardiologists and a 21-percent reduction in other medical visits—roughly consistent with our assumption that the CHF management program would eliminate 90 percent of hospital outpatient department visits and office visits to physicians that are associated with a CHF diagnosis. But the CHF management program itself requires office visits to a physician, so we added 4.5 visits per year for each enrollee.

Table 6.10
Effect of CHF Management on Utilization, Expenditures, and Days Affected[a]

	Under 65	65 and Older	Total	Range of Total	
				Low	High
Population (millions)	0.4	1.0	1.4		
Utilization Measures (millions)					
Inpatient Stays	−0.2[a]	−0.6	−0.7	−0.4	−1.1
Inpatient Nights	−1.1[a]	−4.7	−5.8	−3.5	−8.7
Hosp Outpatient + ER Visits	−0.1[a]	−0.4	−0.5	−0.3	−0.7
Office Visits	−0.6	−2.1	−2.7	−2.7	−2.7
Disease Mgt Visits	1.8	4.7	6.4		
Expenditures ($billions)					
Hospital	−$1.7	−$5.7	−$7.4	−$4.5	−$11.0
Physician	−$0.3	−$0.9	−$1.2	−$0.8	−$1.7
Program Cost	$0.3	$0.7	$1.0	$1.0	$1.0
Rx	$0.1	$0.2	$0.3	$0.5	$0.1
Total	−$1.6	−$5.7	−$7.3	−$3.8	−$11.6
Days Affected (millions)					
Schooldays Lost	0.0	0.0	0.0		
Workdays Lost	−1.8	−1.2	−3.0		
Total Days Abed	−10.8	−27.9	−38.8		
Mortality (thousands)					
Deaths	−17.8	−149.6	−167.4		

NOTES: Detail may not add to total due to rounding.
[a]Total deaths were estimated from 86 observations from the MEPS dataset, 11 for the "Under 65" population and 75 for the "65 and Older" population. All other items were estimated from more than 180 observations. The AHRQ declines to report estimates made from fewer than 100 observations.

Effects on Expenditures. We reduced expenditures reported for ER visits, hospital stays, and outpatient and office visits by the same percentages as we reduced utilization. We then summarized expenditure reductions by recipient. Hospitals receive part of the expenditures from ER visits, inpatient stays, and outpatient visits, and physicians bill separately for the rest. Physicians bear the entire reduction in expenditures on office visits.

We have calculated the program cost as the average cost per person assuming basic HIT, or $718.33 per enrollee per year. We have reported this number separately in Table 6.10, although we suspect that most of it would be paid to physician practices.

Effects on Outcomes. We also estimated the effect of our CHF management program on days spent sick in bed, days lost from school, and days lost from work. As we did for diabetes, we compared the population diagnosed with CHF to a comparison population with the same distribution over sex, age categories, and ethnicities, but without CHF. We found no literature reports of the effect of CHF disease management on workdays lost or days spent sick in bed. If we value these days at the same rates as we did for diabetes, the indirect savings from a comprehensive CHF management program would be $2.36 billion per year.

We have not estimated the short-term effect of CHF management on mortality, but here are some facts from which we can develop a very rough sense of the possibilities. First, of the four diseases we have considered managing, this is the only one for which the literature suggests that management has an effect on short-term mortality. Clarke and Nash (2002) report that the "death rate is 6% during the first year of the program, compared to 19% nationally."

The CDC reports 710,760 deaths from diseases of the heart in 2000, of which 55,704 were from heart failure. The former figure is about 50 percent of the prevalence of CHF found in the MEPS, which agrees with the observation of Jessup and Brozena that symptomatic heart failure has a one-year mortality of 45 percent. But the figure includes many diagnoses in addition to CHF.

If we take 19 percent (from Clarke and Nash) of the prevalence of CHF in the MEPS, we get 271,000 deaths per year. The MEPS shows a total of 219,000 deaths among people with CHF—about 15 percent of people diagnosed with the disease—which agrees pretty well with Clarke and Nash's 19 percent. Reducing these figures from 19 to 6 percent yields a reduction in first-year mortality of 150,000 (13/19ths of MEPS deaths), to 191,000 (13 percent of MEPS's prevalence).

A comparison group from the MEPS without CHF but matched on age, sex, and ethnicity shows 51,000 deaths, for a difference of 167,000. According to the literature, CHF management cuts hospitalizations by about half. Using the same speculative reasoning as for diabetes, we can infer that mortality might be reduced by 84,000 in the short term.

All of this discussion points to a first-year reduction on the order of 100,000 deaths, if everyone with class 3 and class 4 CHF were enrolled in a disease management program such as we described earlier. However, this is only first-year mortality. We have no information about mortality in subsequent years. It is very plausible that disease management adds no more than one year to the life of a person with severe CHF.

Asthma Management

The Population with Asthma

We took a respondent in the trajectory file to have asthma if the pair of a CCC and a 3-digit ICD-9 code in Table 6.11 is associated with that respondent.

The CDC reports that a total of 20 million people had asthma in 2002 and 30.8 million had ever been diagnosed with asthma during their lifetime.[14] The CDC also reports the *prevalence of asthma attacks*—the number of people who have had at least one attack during the previous year—as 12 million people in 2002. From the MEPS, we calculated that 11.7 million people report having asthma, and most (9.1 million) have a medical event (e.g., office visit, prescription) that lists this condition. We would compare the lower figure from the MEPS (9.1 million) with the CDC's attack prevalence (12 million), and we regard the two figures as reasonably close. It is not surprising that the larger number calculated from the MEPS (11.7 million) is well below the CDC's "true" prevalence of the diagnosis (20 million), because respondents with asthma might very well not report it if they did not purchase any prescription drugs for asthma, and never had an office visit, a hospital stay, or a visit to a hospital ER or outpatient department for asthma.

Asthma Management Costs

To construct our model of asthma management costs, we consulted an NPC report that summarizes over 50 studies on asthma management programs (NPC, 2004a) and a similar Center for the Advancement of Health report on asthma (CFAH, 2000), plus an overview of disease management programs by Gillespie (2002). Additional information on asthma disease management design and the time requirements were derived from Krishna et al. (2003), Kelly et al. (1998), and Chan, Callahan, and Moreno (2001) on pediatric asthma; Jowers, Schwartz, and Tinkelman (2000), Burton et al. (2001), and Patel, Welsh, and Foggs (2004) on adult asthma management.

The largest part of any asthma program is education, which teaches patient self-monitoring. Most programs for the general asthmatic population suggest 3 to 6

Table 6.11
MEPS Diagnoses Included in Asthma

CCC	CCC Label	ICD9.3	ICD9.3 Label
128	Asthma	493	ASTHMA*

NOTE: The asterisk is part of the ICD9.3 label. It does not refer to this note.

---

[14] See http://www.cdc.gov/nchs/products/pubs/pubd/hestats/asthma/asthma.htm; accessed on January 2, 2005.

hours of group education (Bolton et al., 1991; Yoon et al., 1993; Kotses et al., 1996; and Wilson et al., 1993); programs for severe asthmatics provide about 10 hours of group education (Allen et al., 1995; Kotses, Bernstein, and Bernstein, 1995; Pettersson et al., 1999). The CFAH report on asthma (2000) suggests that asthma disease management should also "include three to four regular outpatient visits per year to monitor progress and adjust medication and behavior management plans." Rather than initiating regular contacts with the patient, the nurses provide hotline access for the patients with questions and current symptoms, coupled with follow-up. An often-cited feature of an asthma disease management program is a home visit to conduct an environmental assessment in cases in which environmental asthma triggers are suspected.

Guided by a clinician's advice, we assumed that 70 percent of asthmatics have only mild intermittent or mild persistent asthma. These patients need no more than a packet of educational materials ($50 per patient) or perhaps a special website for asthma education. We reserved our asthma management programs for meeting the needs of moderate persistent asthma patients (20 percent) and severe persistent asthma patients (10 percent). Our model thus calculated costs for only the two more-severe categories, as shown in Table 6.12.

Guided by the advice of a clinician, we assumed the ratio of prevalence to annual incidence to be around 7 percent, which we used to weight the costs in the first and subsequent years. If we assumed mild asthmatics will be enrolled, and twice the number of moderate as severe asthmatics, then the average costs are $90.87 per patient per year for basic HIT and $62.83 per patient per year for advanced HIT.

Asthma Management Benefits

Table 6.13 presents our estimates of the effects of our model asthma management program on healthcare utilization, healthcare expenditures, and selected outcomes. We estimated these quantities by generating a table such as Table 6.2 from the MEPS database and applying factors from the published literature. We obtained

Table 6.12
Cost of Asthma Management per Patient per Year

HIT Level	Severity	First Year	Subsequent Years
Basic	Mild	$50.00	$0.00
Basic	Moderate	$392.60	$190.68
Basic	Severe	$783.30	$451.29
Advanced	Mild	$50.00	$0.00
Advanced	Moderate	$217.14	$144.27
Advanced	Severe	$503.16	$311.22

Table 6.13
Effect of Asthma Management on Utilization, Expenditures, and Days Affected[a]

	Under 65	65 and Older	Total	Range of Total Low	Range of Total High
Population (millions)	10.5	1.2	11.7		
Utilization Measures (millions)					
Inpatient Stays	−0.3	−0.1	−0.3	−0.3	−0.4
Inpatient Nights	−1.0	−0.6	−1.6	−1.4	−1.8
Hosp Outpatient + ER Visits	−1.1	−0.1	−1.2	−1.0	−1.3
Office Visits	-9.4	−2.2	−11.6	−10.9	−12.2
Disease Mgt Visits	17.9	2.0	19.9	19.9	19.9
Expenditures ($billions)					
Hospital	−$1.1	−$0.4	−$1.4	−$1.2	−$1.6
Physician	−$1.0	−$0.3	−$1.3	−$1.2	−$1.3
Program Cost	$1.0	$0.1	$1.1	$1.1	$1.1
Rx	$1.2	$0.3	$1.5	$2.9	$0.4
Total	$0.1	−$0.3	−$0.2	$1.6	−$1.5
Days Affected (millions)					
Schooldays Lost	−12.2	0.0	−12.2		
Workdays Lost	−13.9	−0.5	−14.4		
Total Days Abed	−50.4	−8.9	−59.3		
Mortality (thousands)					
Deaths	−13.1	6.2	−6.9		

NOTES: Detail may not add to total due to rounding.
[a]Total deaths were estimated from 34 observations from the MEPS dataset, 12 for the "Under 65" population and 22 for the "65 and Older" population. All other items were estimated from more than 500 observations. The AHRQ declines to report estimates made from fewer than 100 observations.

three values for most factors: low, middle, and high. We used the middle values to estimate the quantities in the first three columns. The last two columns show the range of the "Total" column, calculated using the low and high values for the factors. We make no adjustments for MEPS respondents who might already have been in asthma management programs, which results in an overestimate of both benefits and costs.

Effects on Utilization Measures. Jowers, Schwartz, and Tinkelman (2000) report a reduction in ER visits of 73 to 88 percent; Patel, Welsh, and Foggs (2004), 41 to 43 percent; Kelly et al. (1998), 59 percent; and Zeiger et al. (1991), 50 percent. Reductions in hospitalizations are much more widely documented: Kelly et al. (1998), 74 percent; Mayo, Richman, and Harris (1990), 50 to 70 percent; Yoon et al. (1993), 90 percent (for asthma-related readmissions); Jowers, Schwartz, and Tinkelman (2000), 67 to 88 percent; Patel, Welsh, and Foggs (2004), 54 to 57 percent; and Chan, Callahan, and Moreno (2001), 30 to 40 percent. Overall, the studies on the effects of asthma management report larger reductions in hospitalizations than in ER visits. We assumed that the reduction in asthma-related admissions is about 70 percent for ER visits and 80 percent for asthma-related inpatient admissions. Unlike the other disease management models, for asthma we do not reduce ER visits and hospitalizations that are not associated with an asthma diagnosis.

As we did for diabetes and CHF, we assumed that the asthma management program would eliminate 90 percent of hospital outpatient department or office visits to physicians that are associated with an asthma diagnosis. But the program itself requires office visits to a physician, so we added 1.7 visits per year for each enrollee.

Effects on Expenditures. We reduced expenditures reported for ER visits, hospital stays, and outpatient and office visits by the same percentages as we reduced utilization. We then summarized expenditure reductions by recipient. Hospitals receive part of the expenditures from ER visits, inpatient stays, and outpatient visits, and physicians bill separately for the rest. Physicians bear the entire reduction in expenditures on office visits.

Drug utilization usually increases as a result of asthma disease management—for example, Rossiter et al. (2000) reported a 25-percent increase in utilization of some reliever drugs recommended for asthma. We have used estimates of 15 percent (low), 50 percent (middle), and 100 percent (high).

We calculated the program cost as the average cost per person, assuming basic HIT, or $90.87 per enrollee per year. We have reported this number separately, although we suspect most of it would be paid to physician practices.

Effects on Outcomes. We also estimated the effect of our asthma management program on days spent sick in bed, days lost from school, and days lost from work. As we did for diabetes, we compared the population diagnosed with asthma to a population with the same distribution over sex, age categories, and ethnicities, but without asthma. If we value these days at the same rates as we did for diabetes, the indirect savings from a comprehensive asthma management program would be $5.22 billion per year.

According to the literature, asthma management produces substantial savings for work- and schooldays missed. Jowers, Schwartz, and Tinkelman (2000) report that workdays missed decreased by 67 to 80 percent; Gallefoss and Bakke (2000), 69 percent; Lahdensuo, Haahtela, and Herrala (1996), 40 percent; Kauppinen et al. (2001), 60 percent. Kelly et al. (1998) reported that schooldays missed decreased by 32 percent; Ross, Togger, and Desjardins (1998), 20 percent. Our method yielded reductions of 55 percent in totals days sick in bed and in schooldays missed, and 40 percent in workdays missed.

There is very little mortality from asthma. The CDC data show only about 4,500 deaths attributed to asthma in 2000. The MEPS shows a total of 72,000 deaths of people with asthma, but these are deaths from all causes. An asthma-free comparison group matched on age, sex, and ethnicity shows a total of 65,000 deaths, for a difference of 7,000 deaths, which seems to be in line with the CDC number. We conclude that asthma management has no significant effect on mortality.

COPD Management

The Population with COPD

Chronic obstructive pulmonary disease (COPD) can be defined broadly or narrowly. The Global Initiative for Chronic Obstructive Lung Disease (GOLD), a collaboration between the National Heart, Lung, and Blood Institute (NHLBI) and the World Health Organization (WHO) (GOLD, 2004), defines *COPD* as

> a disease state characterized by airflow limitation that is not fully reversible. The airflow limitation is usually both progressive and associated with an abnormal inflammatory response of the lungs to noxious particles or gases.

The NHLBI defines it as including chronic bronchitis, chronic obstructive bronchitis, emphysema, or combinations of these conditions.[15] We captured this definition by including the diagnostic codes shown in Table 6.14.

According to the NHLBI, 12.1 million Americans are living with a diagnosis of COPD, including 9.2 million with chronic bronchitis, 2 million with emphysema, and 0.9 million with both. We calculated from the MEPS that 1.9 million people have one or both of these diagnoses. However, the MEPS shows 12.5 million people with any diagnosis of bronchitis, including the chronic form that we have included in

Table 6.14
MEPS Diagnoses Included in COPD

CCC	CCC Label	ICD9.3	ICD9.3 Label
127	Chronic obstructive pulmonary disease and bronchiectasis	491	CHRONIC BRONCHITIS*
		492	EMPHYSEMA*

NOTE: The asterisk is part of the ICD9.3 label. It does not refer to this note.

---

[15] See http://www.nhlbi.nih.gov; accessed on December 31, 2004.

our definition of the condition, plus Bronchitis NOS (not otherwise specified). The MEPS can be made to agree with the figure reported by the NHLBI if most MEPS respondents with Bronchitis NOS are assumed to have the chronic form of the disease.

COPD Management Costs

To construct our model of COPD management costs, we consulted an NPC report (NPC, 2003), plus descriptions of COPD programs from Bourbeau et al. (2003) and Zajac (2002). Since smoking is the single most important risk factor of COPD, smoking cessation becomes a major goal of COPD management (Hunter and King, 2001). In our model, we assumed that smokers make two visits to the smoking-cessation specialist in the first year, and one visit in subsequent years, in addition to receiving regular advice from the physician and a nurse during education activities. Home visits by a nurse might be a necessary element of COPD management for assessment, primary education, or exercise training, given that this condition is debilitating and prevails among the elderly.

We separated people with COPD into two severity groups: moderate (two-thirds) and severe (one-third). Table 6.15 shows the costs per patient per year.

We assumed that one-third of patients in the program will be in their first year and two-thirds in a subsequent year, which leads to average costs of the program of $486.80 per patient per year with basic HIT and $329.74 per patient per year with advanced HIT.

COPD Management Benefits

Table 6.16 presents our estimates of the effects of our model COPD management program on healthcare utilization, healthcare expenditures, and selected outcomes. We estimated these quantities by generating a table such as Table 6.2 from the MEPS database and applying factors from the published literature. We obtained

Table 6.15
Cost of COPD Management per Patient per Year

HIT Level	Severity	First Year	Subsequent Years
Basic	Moderate	$628.79	$298.88
Basic	Severe	$910.72	$509.57
Advanced	Moderate	$392.91	$236.88
Advanced	Severe	$586.32	$324.45

Table 6.16
Effect of COPD Management on Utilization, Expenditures, and Outcomes[a]

	Under 65	65 and Older	Total	Range of Total	
				Low	High
Population (millions)	0.9	1.0	1.9		
Utilization Measures (millions)					
Inpatient Stays	−0.1	−0.3	−0.4	−0.2	−0.5
Inpatient Nights	−0.7	−1.7	−2.5	−1.5	−3.1
Hosp Outpatient + ER Visits	−0.2	−0.2	−0.4	−0.2	−0.5
Office Visits	−1.2	−1.7	−2.9	−2.7	−3.0
Disease Mgt Visits	3.5	4.1	7.6		
Expenditures ($billions)					
Hospital	−$0.9	−$2.0	−$2.8	−$1.7	−$3.6
Physician	−$0.2	−$0.4	−$0.7	−$0.5	−$0.8
Program Cost	$0.4	$0.5	$0.9	$0.9	$0.9
Rx	$0.1	$0.1	$0.2	$0.2	$0.1
Total	−$0.6	−$1.8	−$2.4	−$1.0	−$3.4
Days Affected (millions)					
Schooldays Lost	−0.1	0.0	−0.1		
Workdays Lost	−2.2	0.2	−1.9		
Total Days Abed	−14.4	−21.0	−35.5		
Mortality (thousands)					
Deaths	−19.9	−87.4	−107.3		

NOTES: Detail may not add to total due to rounding.
[a]Total deaths were estimated from 49 observations from the MEPS dataset, 13 for the "Under 65" population and 36 for the "65 and Older" population. All other items were estimated from more than 350 observations. The AHRQ declines to report estimates made from fewer than 100 observations.

three values for most factors: low, middle, and high. We used the middle values to estimate the quantities in the first three columns. The last two columns show the range of the "Total" column, calculated using the low and high values for the factors. We make no adjustments for MEPS respondents who might already have been in COPD management programs, which results in an overestimate of both benefits and costs.

Effects on Utilization Measures. Only a few articles have measured the effect of COPD disease management on utilization. Bourbeau et al. (2003) report reductions in ER visits of 40 percent for COPD and 20 percent for other problems. Reductions in hospitalizations are reported in the following range: 40 percent for COPD and 60 percent for other problems (Bourbeau et al., 2003); 13 to 26 percent by Zajac

(2002); and 42 percent by Stothard and Brewer (2001). We have used 20, 35, and 45 percent for ER visits and 25, 40, and 50 percent for inpatient stays.

As with the other three diseases, we assumed that the COPD management program would eliminate 90 percent of hospital outpatient department or office visits to physicians that are associated with a COPD diagnosis. But the program itself requires office visits to a physician, so we added 1.7 visits per year for each enrollee. This assumption seems reasonable when compared with the result reported by Gallefoss and Bakke (2000), an 85-percent reduction in physician visits as a result of a COPD management program.

Effects on Expenditures. We reduced expenditures reported for ER visits, hospital stays, and outpatient and office visits by the same percentages as we reduced utilization. We then summarized expenditure reductions by recipient. Hospitals receive part of the expenditures from ER visits, inpatient stays, and outpatient visits, and physicians bill separately for the rest. Physicians bear the entire reduction in expenditures on office visits.

We calculated the program cost as the average cost per person, assuming basic HIT, or $486.80 per enrollee per year. We have reported this number separately, although we suspect that most of it would be paid to physician practices.

Most studies (e.g., Gallefoss and Bakke, 2002; Stothard and Brewer, 2001) report a reduction in the utilization of rescue medications. We assumed a reduction of 20 percent, with a range from 10 to 30 percent.

Effects on Outcomes. We also estimated the effect of our COPD management program on days spent sick in bed, days lost from school, and days lost from work. As we did for diabetes, we compared the population diagnosed with COPD to a matched population with the same distribution over sex, age categories, and ethnicities, but without COPD. Overall, we estimated that enrollment in the program should reduce total days abed by 74 percent and workdays missed by 34 percent. Gallefoss and Bakke (2000) report a 95-percent reduction in workdays lost. If we value these days at the same rates as we did for diabetes, the indirect savings from a comprehensive COPD management program would be $2.05 billion per year.

We have not estimated the short-term effect of COPD management on mortality, but here are some speculations. The CDC shows 17,867 deaths from emphysema or chronic bronchitis—our definition of COPD—in 2000. The MEPS shows a total of 149,000 deaths among people with COPD. A matched comparison group without COPD shows only 42,000 deaths, for a difference of 107,000. This is much larger than the CDC number. But remember that CDC is reporting the number of death certificates with emphysema or chronic bronchitis recorded as the main cause of death. Many of these deaths might be attributed to something else.

There is certainly scope for disease management to delay deaths of people with COPD. The literature suggests that disease management reduces inpatient stays by 60 percent (to 40 percent of the unmanaged rate). If all the deaths occurred in the hospital, and if the fraction of inpatient stays resulting in death remained the same, the mortality rate should drop in the short term by 60 percent, or something on the order of 64,000 (60 percent of 107,000) to 89,000 (60 percent of 149,000) deaths. We know of no published evidence supporting these assumptions, but they seem as plausible as any others. However, no one seems to have claimed a mortality reduction as one of the benefits of COPD management.

Aligning and Projecting Effects of the Four Disease-Management Programs

In Chapter Three, we found that utilization and expenditure measures in the MEPS need to be adjusted so that they are aligned with the provider-based data sources that are generally considered to be more authoritative. In addition, to project the effects of these programs from the year 2000 into future years, we must adjust them for demographic changes and further inflate expenditures. Table 6.17 shows the results of these calculations.

Table 6.17
Combined, Aligned, and Projected Effects of the Four Disease-Management Programs
(assuming 100-percent participation)

Year	Raw MEPS 2000	MEPS Aligned with Authoritative Sources				
		2000	2005	2010	2015	2020
Population (millions)	26.6	26.6	28.3	30.2	32.4	34.7
Utilization Measures (millions)						
Inpatient Stays	−3.6	−3.6	−3.9	−4.3	−4.7	−5.3
Inpatient Nights	−26.3	−26.3	−28.6	−31.3	−34.7	−38.7
Hosp Outpatient + ER Visits	−4.9	−9.0	−14.6	−16.1	−17.9	−19.6
Office Visits	−46.7	−46.7	−51.2	−56.0	−61.7	−67.6
Disease Mgt Visits	80.0	80.0	86.0	92.9	100.8	109.0
Expenditures ($billions)						
Hospital	−$30.1	−$36.5	−$52.9	−$73.4	−$100.3	−$137.7
Physician	−$8.5	−$13.1	−$19.2	−$28.2	−$40.4	−$57.9
Program Cost	$8.5	$8.5	$12.5	$18.1	$25.7	$36.4
Rx	$1.9	$1.9	$3.6	$6.1	$9.5	$14.8
Total	−$28.3	−$39.2	−$56.1	−$77.3	−$105.5	−$144.5
Days Affected (millions)						
Schooldays Lost	−12.9	−12.9	−13.1	−13.2	−13.4	−13.8
Workdays Lost	−28.2	−28.2	−29.8	−31.1	−31.9	−32.0
Total Days Abed	−244.6	−244.6	−267.6	−291.6	−317.8	−346.0

The first column is simply the sum of the "Total" columns of the effects tables for the four individual programs (Tables 6.6, 6.10, 6.13, and 6.16). The second column aligns the utilization measures with the more-authoritative National Hospital Ambulatory Medical Care Survey (NHAMCS), and the expenditures with the more-authoritative NHE, as described in Chapter Three. For subsequent columns, we estimated effects for future years by the same methods as for the first column, but using the person-weights for future years (see Chapter Two) rather than for the year 2000. Then we adjusted utilization and expenditures so that they were aligned with the more-authoritative sources and inflated the expenditures from 2000 to each of the future years, using the escalation factors from Table 3.23.

Because some people have multiple chronic conditions, so that adding the effects involves some double-counting, it is slightly incorrect to add effects from the four individual programs. To get an idea how large an error such double-counting introduced, we compared the number of people in the trajectory file that have one or more of these four conditions with the sum of the numbers that have each of the four individual conditions. The first number is over 93 percent of the second, so our estimates should be about 7 percent too large.

It may be worthwhile to review just what question Table 6.17 answers: "Suppose we were able to observe two versions of history. In one version, all eligible people are enrolled in the appropriate one of the four disease-management programs. In the other version, nobody is enrolled. What difference would data collected in the years 2000, 2005, 2010, 2015, and 2020 show between the two versions of history?" The first column is our answer to this question for data from the MEPS of the year 2000. The subsequent columns contain our answers for utilization data from the Nationwide Inpatient Sample (NIS), the National Ambulatory Medical Care Survey (NAMCS), and NHAMCS, for expenditures from the NHE, and for health outcomes from the MEPS.

We shifted our perspective from the MEPS to the other data sources, because the other sources are considered to be more accurate. We projected results into the future because it would take years to implement the disease management programs. But having made both of these adjustments, we learned little that we could not see from the unadjusted MEPS-based estimates from the year 2000. Utilization and outcomes grow in future years as the population grows and ages. Expenditures grow due to both population changes and inflation. Our estimates of the effects of disease management grow in proportion.

CHAPTER SEVEN

Estimating Long-Term Effects of Healthy Behavior on Population Health Status and Healthcare

James H. Bigelow, Ph.D., Constance Fung, M.D., and Jason Wang, M.D.

Introduction

Here, we estimate the maximum effects that might flow from a four-step program of lifestyle change and long-term management of silent conditions, such as hypertension and high cholesterol. The steps are as follows:

1. Everybody adopts the combination of lifestyle changes and (as necessary) medication use that best promotes good health.
2. These changes reduce the incidence of a number of chronic medical conditions.
3. Over time, the reduction in the incidence of each condition results in a reduction in the prevalence of each condition.
4. Because these conditions are less prevalent, utilization of and expenditures on healthcare decline, and measures of health status improve.

Although it may seem overly optimistic to think that a large fraction of the population could be persuaded to adopt healthy habits, we believe that Health Information Technology (HIT) can play a role in such adoption (step 1). Large numbers of us have habits that ill serve our health, some smoking, others overeating, and many not exercising. However, people are capable of changing their behavior. For example, between 1965 and 2001, the fraction of people over 18 who smoke dropped from 42 percent to 23 percent (NCHS, 2003). Step 1 is large enough by itself that we devote a separate chapter, Chapter Eight, to discussing it.

In this chapter, we suppose that step 1 has been accomplished, and we estimate its long-term effects as outlined in steps 2, 3, and 4. The effects we estimate are those listed in steps 3 and 4—prevalence of selected diseases, healthcare utilization, healthcare expenditures, and population health status.

We embedded our estimates in the world of 2000, which is the world described by the trajectory file we assembled from the Medical Expenditure Panel Survey (MEPS) (see Chapter Two). Thus, we assumed the same population, the same technology, and the same propensities to seek medical attention that gave rise to our database. In short, we are asking what healthcare in 2000 might have looked like if everybody alive at that time had lived a healthy life (as defined in step 1 above) from birth to 2000. This approach has the advantage of obviating the need to generate scenarios for the future healthcare system. But it has the disadvantage of ignoring the fact that if everybody adopted healthier habits, they would live longer. During those extra years of life, they would surely consume healthcare resources. Indeed, it has been suggested that during those extra years, they would acquire costly conditions, such as Alzheimer's disease, and might end up consuming more healthcare resources than if they had retained their unhealthy habits (Maeder, 2001).

Lack of time and resources prevented us from pursuing this issue. We agree that people will continue to consume healthcare during their extra years, but we think it is unduly pessimistic to assume that they will get so sick and feeble in those years as to wipe out the savings accrued during the years they would have lived anyway. Moreover, those extra years ought to be worth something.

In the remainder of this chapter, we first define the medical conditions whose incidences we will change. Next, we present some findings from the literature that suggest how large a reduction in incidences we should consider. Then we discuss our methodology for representing how changing incidences alter the trajectory database. Fourth, we estimate the effects of these incidence changes on healthcare utilization, healthcare expenditures, and population health status. These estimates assume that 100 percent of the population participates in step 1. Fifth, we discuss how these estimates can be combined with the disease management results from Chapter Six and how they can be adjusted to reflect less than 100-percent participation. Sixth, we use the methods of Chapter Three to align the expenditure results with the more-authoritative National Health Expenditures (NHE), and we project the results to future years.

Target Conditions

We consider changes to the incidence of selected cardiovascular conditions (hypertension, hyperlipidemia, coronary artery disease/acute myocardial infarction (AMI), congestive heart failure (CHF), cerebrovascular disease/stroke, and other heart diseases), diabetes and its complications (retinopathy, neuropathy, lower extremity foot ulcers and amputations, kidney diseases, and heart diseases), chronic obstructive pulmonary disease (COPD) (emphysema and chronic bronchitis), and the cancers most strongly associated with smoking (cancers of the bronchus and lung, cancers of the head and neck, cancer of the esophagus, and other respiratory and intrathoracic cancers). Table 7.1 lists the MEPS diagnoses (i.e., pairs of Clinical Classification Code [CCC] codes and 3-digit *International Classification of Diseases,* Revision 9 [ICD-9] codes) that we have included in each condition.

Table 7.1
MEPS Diagnoses Included in Target Conditions

CCC	CCC Label	ICD9.3	ICD9.3 Label
		Diabetes	
049	Diabetes mellitus without complication	250	DIABETES MELLITUS*
		790	ABNORMAL BLOOD FINDINGS*
		791	ABNORMAL URINE FINDINGS*
050	Diabetes mellitus with complications	250	DIABETES MELLITUS*
		Chronic Renal Failure	
158	Chronic renal failure	585	CHRONIC RENAL FAILURE
		792	ABN FIND-OTH BODY SUBST*
		V42	ORGAN TRANSPLANT STATUS*
		V45	OTH POSTSURGICAL STATES*
		V56	DIALYSIS ENCOUNTER*
		Lower Limb Involvement	
114	Peripheral and visceral atherosclerosis	440	ATHEROSCLEROSIS*
199	Chronic ulcer of skin	707	CHRONIC ULCER OF SKIN*
211	Other connective tissue disease	V49	LIMB PROBLEM/PROBLEM NEC*
		Retinopathy	
087	Retinal detachments, defects, vascular occlusion, and retinopathy	362	RETINAL DISORDERS NEC*
		Neuropathy	
095	Other nervous system disorders	337	AUTONOMIC NERVE DISORDER*
		355	MONONEURITIS LEG*
		Hypertension	
098	Essential hypertension	401	ESSENTIAL HYPERTENSION*
099	Hypertension with complications and secondary hypertension	401	ESSENTIAL HYPERTENSION*
		402	HYPERTENSIVE HEART DIS*
		403	HYPERTENSIVE RENAL DIS*
		459	OTH CIRCULATORY DISEASE*

Table 7.1—Continued

CCC	CCC Label	ICD9.3	ICD9.3 Label
		Hyperlipidemia	
053	Disorders of lipid metabolism	272	DIS OF LIPOID METABOLISM*
		Coronary Artery Disease	
100	Acute myocardial infarction	410	ACUTE MYOCARDIAL INFARCT*
101	Coronary atherosclerosis and other heart disease	411	OTH AC ISCHEMIC HRT DIS*
		412	OLD MYOCARDIAL INFARCT
		413	ANGINA PECTORIS*
		414	OTH CHR ISCHEMIC HRT DIS*
		V45	OTH POSTSURGICAL STATES*
		Cerebrovascular Disease/Stroke	
109	Acute cerebrovascular disease	430	SUBARACHNOID HEMORRHAGE
		431	INTRACEREBRAL HEMORRHAGE
		432	INTRACRANIAL HEM NEC/NOS*
		434	CEREBRAL ARTERY OCCLUS*
		436	CVA
		437	OTH CEREBROVASC DISEASE*
110	Occlusion or stenosis of precerebral arteries	433	PRECEREBRAL OCCLUSION*
112	Transient cerebral ischemia	435	TRANSIENT CEREB ISCHEMIA*
113	Late effects of cerebrovascular disease	438	LATE EFF CEREBROVASC DIS*
		Heart Failure	
108	Congestive heart failure, nonhypertensive	428	HEART FAILURE*
		Other Heart Diseases	
096	Heart valve disorders	394	DISEASES OF MITRAL VALVE*
		397	ENDOCARDIAL DISEASE NEC*
		424	OTH ENDOCARDIAL DISEASE*
		785	CARDIOVASCULAR SYS SYMP*
		V42	ORGAN TRANSPLANT STATUS*
		V43	ORGAN REPLACEMENT NEC*
097	Peri-, endo-, and myocarditis, cardiomyopathy (except that caused by tuberculosis or sexually transmitted disease)	139	LATE EFFECT INFECT NEC*
		391	RHEUM FEV W HEART INVOLV*
		398	OTH RHEUMATIC HEART DIS*
		420	ACUTE PERICARDITIS*
		422	ACUTE MYOCARDITIS*
		423	OTH PERICARDIAL DISEASE*

Table 7.1—Continued

CCC	CCC Label	ICD9.3	ICD9.3 Label
	Other Heart Diseases—Continued		
		425	CARDIOMYOPATHY*
		429	ILL-DEFINED HEART DIS*
102	Nonspecific chest pain	786	RESP SYS/OTH CHEST SYMP*
103	Pulmonary heart disease	415	ACUTE PULMONARY HRT DIS*
		416	CHR PULMONARY HEART DIS*
104	Other and ill-defined heart disease	414	OTH CHR ISCHEMIC HRT DIS*
		429	ILL-DEFINED HEART DIS*
105	Conduction disorders	426	CONDUCTION DISORDERS*
		V45	OTH POSTSURGICAL STATES*
		V53	ADJUSTMENT OF OTH DEVICE*
106	Cardiac dysrhythmias	427	CARDIAC DYSRHYTHMIAS*
		785	CARDIOVASCULAR SYS SYMP*
107	Cardiac arrest and ventricular fibrillation	427	CARDIAC DYSRHYTHMIAS*
	COPD		
127	Chronic obstructive pulmonary disease and bronchiectasis	491	CHRONIC BRONCHITIS*
		492	EMPHYSEMA*
	Smoking-Related Cancers		
011	Cancer of head and neck	140	MALIGNANT NEOPLASM LIP*
		141	MALIG NEO TONGUE*
		142	MAL NEO MAJOR SALIVARY*
		143	MALIG NEOPLASM GUM*
		144	MAL NEOPLASM FLOOR MOUTH*
		145	MALIG NEO MOUTH NEC/NOS*
		146	MALIG NEO OROPHARYNX*
		147	MAL NEOPLASM NASOPHARYN*
		148	MAL NEOPLASM PHARYNX*
		149	OTH MALIG NEO OROPHARYNX*
		160	MAL NEO NASAL CAV/SINUS*
		161	MALIGNANT NEO LARYNX*
		195	MAL NEO OTH/ILL-DEF SITE*
		199	MALIGNANT NEOPLASM NOS*
		230	CA IN SITU ORAL CAV/PHAR
		231	CA IN SITU LARYNX-*/
		V10	HX OF MALIGNANT NEOPLASM*
012	Cancer of esophagus	150	MALIGNANT NEO ESOPHAGUS*
		230	CA IN SITU ESOPHAGUS-*/
		V10	HX OF MALIGNANT NEOPLASM*

Table 7.1—Continued

CCC	CCC Label	ICD9.3	ICD9.3 Label
019	Cancer of bronchus, lung	162	MAL NEO TRACHEA/LUNG*
		231	CA IN SITU BRONCHUS/LUNG-*/
		V10	HX-BRONCHOGENIC MALIGNAN
020	Cancer, other respiratory and intrathoracic	162	MALIGNANT NEO TRACHEA
		163	MALIG NEOPL PLEURA
		165	MAL NEO RESP SYSTEM
		231	CA IN SITU RESP SYS
		V10	HX OF MALIGNANT NEOPLASM*
		147	MAL NEOPLASM NASOPHARYN*

NOTES: The asterisk is part of the ICD9.3 label. It does not refer to this note.
NEC = not elsewhere considered.
NOS = not otherwise specified.

Potential Reductions in the Incidences of Target Conditions

The literature suggests that lifestyle changes and medications can reduce the incidence of each of these conditions substantially. As shown in Table 7.2, such measures can reduce stroke, coronary artery disease/acute myocardial infarction (CAD/AMI), diabetes, and complications of diabetes to as little as 40 percent of their baseline levels. Smoking cessation can reduce the incidence of COPD and smoking-related cancers. Combinations of diet, exercise, weight control, and medications can control hypertension and hyperlipidemia, which are risk factors for more-serious cardiovascular conditions. Weight control can reduce the incidence of diabetes and its complications. Moreover, most of our target conditions are affected by more than one intervention, as shown in the Framingham Heart Study (e.g., Wilson et al., 1998).[1] For simplicity, we evaluated the effects of a hypothetical package of lifestyle and other changes that reduces the incidence of each of our target conditions to 40 percent of its baseline value.

Long-Term Effect on Prevalence

The immediate effects of interventions are to reduce the *incidences* of these conditions; in the longer term, they reduce *prevalences*. The *incidence* of a condition

---

[1] Medical algorithms have been collected at http://www.medalreg.com. Among them are several from the Framingham Heart Study, including an earlier version of Wilson et al. (1998), a heart-failure predictor, and a stroke-risk predictor. All estimate the probability of an outcome based on multiple risk factors.

Table 7.2
Some Incidence Reductions Found in the Literature

Prevention Measure	Incidence Ratio
Stroke (Bronner, Kanter, and Manson, 1995)	
Diastolic blood pressure (BP) decrease 5-6 mmHg	0.58
Systolic BP decrease 11 mmg	0.64
Smoking cessation	0.65
Physically active life style	0.70
CAD/AMI (Rich-Edwards et al., 1995)	
Smoking cessation	0.50
Every 1% reduction in serum cholesterol	0.98
Treatment of hypertension (use diastolic)	0.84
Treatment of isolated systolic hypertension	0.75
Small to moderate daily alcohol vs. no intake	0.50
At ideal weight vs. obese women	0.53
Physical activity vs. sedentary	0.50
Diabetes (Chiasson et al., 2003; Diabetes Prevention Research Group, 2002)	
Weight reduction and physical activities	0.42
Metformin	0.69
Acarbose	0.75
Diabetes Complications (Chiasson et al., 2003; Clark and Lee, 1995; Diabetes Control and Complications Trial Research Group, 1993)	
Intensive blood glucose reduction to normal value reduces retinopathy	0.50
Photocoagulation reduces blindness in 20 years	0.50
Intensive blood-glucose reduction to normal value reduces albuminuria	0.40
Anglotensin-converting enzyme (ACE) inhibitors reduce end-stage renal disease	0.50
Acarbose reduces CAD/AMI	0.51
Smoking-Related Cancers (American Cancer Society, 2004)	
Male smokers are 20 times more likely than nonsmokers to develop lung cancer	0.05

is the number of new cases in a given year divided by the population at risk; the *prevalence* of a condition is the inventory of cases at a given time divided by the total number of persons in the population at the time. If we assume that the people at risk are the people who do not have the condition then the odds of having the condition (the ratio of those who have it to those who do not) should be proportional to the incidence.

To see this, let us provide terms for each definition:

Incid = incidence of the disease

P_{rev} = prevalence of the disease

P_{tot} = total population

P_{risk} = population at risk (=population without the disease)

T_{surv} = average time a case of the disease persists.

Then we calculate the rate at which people join the group with the disease, as follows:

$$P_{rev} \times P_{tot} = \text{Incid} \times P_{risk} \times T_{surv} \qquad (7.1)$$

That is, the number of people with the disease ($P_{rev} \times P_{tot}$) equals the rate at which people join the group with the disease (Incid $\times P_{risk}$) multiplied by the time a person with the disease remains in the population (T_{surv}). Dividing both sides by P_{risk} yields the expression for odds on the left-hand side and something proportional to incidence on the right-hand side:

$$\text{Odds} = \frac{P \times P}{P} = \text{Incid} \times T \qquad (7.2)$$

The Algorithm

We used this simple equation to adjust the prevalence of a condition to reflect a change in the odds, as the following short example shows. We start with a baseline population containing 100,000 people in total, of whom 20,000 have the condition. We wish to reduce the incidence rate I to 40 percent of its baseline value. Table 7.3 shows the steps we follow to do so.

The first column shows the distribution of the baseline population between those who have the condition and those who do not. In the second column, we scaled back the number of people with the condition to 40 percent of the baseline value (from 20,000 to 8,000), which reduces the total population from 100,000 to 88,000. To restore the population to its baseline size, we multiplied the numbers of people in column 2 by the ratio (100,000/88,000). The result is column 3, the renormalized population—the population we take to represent the long-term effect of the 40-percent reduction in incidence. The odds of having the condition—the ratio of the

Table 7.3
Steps in Adjusting Prevalences

Category of People	Baseline	Scaled to 40%	Renormalized
With condition	20,000	8,000	9,091
Without condition	80,000	80,000	90,909
Total	100,000	88,000	100,000

population with the condition to the population without the condition—have dropped to 40 percent of the baseline value (the value in column 1), from 25 percent to 10 percent.

Many people have multiple conditions, so reducing the prevalence of one condition will affect the number of people who have another. How do we model these interaction effects?

Table 7.4 shows a short example of how we simultaneously adjusted the prevalences of two conditions, labeled A and B. We wished to reduce the odds of each condition to 40 percent of its baseline value. As in the earlier, one-condition example, we used a scale factor of 1.0 for the population that has neither condition and 0.4 for the populations that have exactly one condition. We used a factor of 0.16 (=0.4×0.4) for the population that has both conditions to ensure that all the conditional odds are reduced to 40 percent of their baseline values.

Thus, among all people with condition B, the odds that a person has condition A are reduced from 0.5 to 0.2 (check the ratios of row 4 to row 3 entries). But the two conditions are not statistically independent (having one makes it more likely that a person has the other), so it is impossible to adjust the populations so that both the conditional odds and the overall odds are reduced to 40 percent of baseline values. If the two conditions are independent, then the adjustment described here does reduce the overall odds to 40 percent of baseline.

There is one additional complication. Changing the prevalence of a condition should not alter the age, sex, or ethnic distribution of the population. We therefore separated the people in our analysis dataset into categories by sex, age, and ethnicity. We applied the procedure, as described, to each category individually, thus ensuring that the population totals within each category remain as they are in the baseline.

This procedure generalizes easily to any number of conditions. For example, if we let

w_j = person-weight associated with respondent j in the trajectory file

cat_j = category to which respondent j belongs

$$\text{cond}_{ij} = \begin{cases} 1 & \text{if respondent } j \text{ has condition } i \\ 0 & \text{otherwise} \end{cases}$$

λ_i = scaling factor for incidence of condition i

w'_j = revised person-weight for respondent j

then the revised weights are calculated as

$$w'_j = \left(w_j \cdot \prod_i \lambda_i^{\text{cond}_{ij}} \right) \left(\frac{\sum_{\{k \mid \text{cat}_k = \text{cat}_j\}} w_k}{\sum_{\{k \mid \text{cat}_k = \text{cat}_j\}} w_k \cdot \prod_i \lambda_i^{\text{cond}_{ik}}} \right) \tag{7.3}$$

Equation (7.3) is actually quite simple. First, we specified a scale factor λ_i for each condition. We have used 0.4 in our examples, any value could be chosen.[2] Then, we scaled the weight for each respondent by the product of the scale factors for those conditions (using a factor 1.0 for people with no conditions). Finally, we renormalized the population so that the population in each category has the same total size as the baseline.

Table 7.4
Adjusting Prevalences of Multiple Conditions

Category	Scale Factor	Baseline	Scaled	Renormalized
Not A, not B	1.00	60,000	60,000	81,521
A, not B	0.40	10,000	4,000	5,435
B, not A	0.40	20,000	8,000	10,870
A and B	0.16	10,000	1,600	2,174
Total		100,000	73,600	100,000

---

[2] Even values larger than 1.0 are allowed. Using a factor greater than 1.0 could represent the increase in diabetes prevalence that many people expect, for example.

Our Algorithm Is Flexible . . .

The algorithm "controls for" categories, meaning that it makes sure that the population in a category remains the same after the person-weights are revised. We have controlled for age, sex, and ethnicity by defining the categories of respondents in terms of age, sex, and ethnicity. We have 66 categories, including two sexes (F and M), 11 age ranges (<1, 1–4, 5–14, 15–24, 25–34, 35–44, 45–54, 55–64, 65–74, 75–84, and 85+), and three ethnicities (Hispanic, black but not Hispanic, and other). The categories can be based on any combination of respondent characteristics, such as the educational attainment of respondents. As with age, sex, and ethnicity, changing the incidences of the conditions would not affect the educational attainment of respondents. In that case, what would be controlled for—i.e., what the categories would be defined in terms of—would be educational attainment, as well as age, sex, and ethnicity.

The algorithm adjusts the person-weight of each respondent according to the conditions that respondent has. We have defined the conditions according to diagnoses reported in the MEPS. But one can define conditions according to any respondent characteristics. For example, we ran some preliminary experiments in which we defined conditions based on health insurance coverage. The algorithm then reduces the number of people who have little or no insurance coverage and replaces them with people who have good coverage.

. . . But It Has Shortcomings

Clearly, our algorithm ignores a plethora of factors. Instead of just scaling prevalences as described, we could have constructed a model that described the disease progression in some detail. Such a model could allow for different incidence rates by age, different survival times by age of onset, and perhaps other details. Markov models have the flexibility to include the factors just mentioned, and they are commonly used to describe chronic disease progression (Sonnenberg and Beck, 1993). For example, the CDC Diabetes Cost-Effectiveness Group (2002) created a series of Markov models to describe the way complications develop in diabetes, and it used the model to estimate the cost-effectiveness of various interventions (Earnshaw et al., 2002; Hoerger et al., 2004). Weinstein et al. (1987) constructed a Markov model to forecast coronary heart disease and its sequelae; Phillips et al. (2000) used that model to estimate the benefits of beta-blockers after AMI. Homer et al. (2003) constructed their own Markov models of diabetes and heart failure to study chronic illness care.[3]

A Markov model could also estimate the effect that changing incidences of conditions would have on the size and age distribution of the population. It does not

---

[3] Markov models are sometimes solved analytically, but more often they serve as the basis for simulations. All the citations given here used simulations.

ignore the fact that if everybody adopted healthier habits, they would live longer and would continue to consume healthcare resources during those extra years of life.[4]

But a Markov model that took into account different incidence rates and survival times for people of different ages would require a considerable amount of data to populate it. The data requirements would be substantial, even for a model dealing with a single condition, and they grow exponentially as more conditions are added.[5] The existing knowledge base is not adequate to provide reliable data at this level of detail, so there is no guarantee that results from a detailed model will be better than the results from our simple algorithm.

The results we obtained should be viewed as very rough and uncertain. As you will see, we think that the long-term effects of the interventions outlined in step 1 (at the outset of this chapter) could be enormous—if everybody adopted them—enough to be worth pursuing.

The Effects

Tables 7.5 and 7.6 show the results (more detail can be found in the Excel file I0D14mlt40.xls, available at http://www.rand.org/publications/MG/MG408 and on the CD included with printed copies of this monograph. Again, we assumed that 100 percent of the population participates in the program. The total expenditures captured in the MEPS file decline by over 20 percent.

Note in Table 7.6 that many of the benefits are divided quite evenly between the under-65 population and the 65-and-older population, despite the fact that the 65-and-over population is so much smaller (13 percent of the total). Chronic diseases are, by and large, diseases of the elderly, which implies that a large fraction of the long-term expenditure reductions due to prevention and management of silent conditions will accrue to Medicare. Yet, to realize these benefits, people should begin participating in these programs as relatively young adults.[6]

---

[4] If we had a model that estimated the postintervention population size and age distribution, we could use its estimates to obtain population totals by category. These totals would replace the category totals in Equation (7.3), which we calculated from the MEPS.

[5] When multiple conditions are involved, they are generally treated as independent, thereby allowing each condition to be treated in a separate model; the results are combined after the fact. See, for example, the Markov models of diabetes complications cited earlier.

[6] In the trajectory file, over half of the people with diabetes, hypertension, or hyperlipidemia are under 65. One in eight is under 45. People should begin participating before they are likely to acquire these conditions.

Table 7.5
Long-Term Effects on Utilization, Expenditures, and Selected Outcomes of a 60-Percent Reduction in Odds of Target Conditions

	Baseline	Reduced Incidence	Delta	Percentage Saved
Utilization Measures (millions)				
Inpatient Stays	28.2	21.1	-7.1	–25.3%
Inpatient Nights	161.4	112.2	–49.2	–30.5%
Hosp Outpatient + ER Visits	93.7	81.2	–12.5	–13.4%
Office Visits	890.2	772.2	–118.0	–13.3%
Expenditures ($billions)				
Hospital	$251.2	$179.6	–$71.7	–28.5%
Physician	$147.6	$124.5	–$23.1	–15.6%
Rx	$94.1	$64.5	–$29.6	–31.5%
Other	$141.0	$126.7	–$14.3	–10.2%
Total	$634.0	$495.3	–$138.7	–21.9%
Days Affected (millions)				
Schooldays Lost	175.6	174.0	–1.6	–0.9%
Workdays Lost	623.4	581.6	–41.9	–6.7%
Total Days Abed	1,332.2	1,075.0	–257.3	–19.3%
Mortality (thousands)				
Deaths	2,067.7	1,667.9	–399.8	–19.3%

Table 7.7 shows the effect of our algorithm on prevalence. As explained earlier in this chapter, reducing the odds of having each of the target conditions by 60 percent will not, in general, reduce the prevalences by 60 percent.

Next, we compared our estimates of these effects to estimates available from the literature. The Centers for Disease Control and Prevention (CDC) (2003) asserts that cardiovascular disease/stroke, diabetes, and smoking-related illnesses have the economic costs shown in Table 7.8.

These costs are substantially higher than the total savings of $139 billion that we estimated, but making certain adjustments narrows the gap. First, cardiovascular diseases and stroke are complications of diabetes, and smoking is a risk factor for cardiovascular diseases and stroke. Thus some double-counting is occurring in the CDC numbers. Second, as explained in Chapter Three, the MEPS contains only part of the total expenditures on healthcare and should be inflated by about 32 percent. Third, the effects in Table 7.5 correspond to a substantial reduction in the prevalence of our target chronic conditions, but not to their total elimination. The CDC numbers should be scaled back to reflect this reduction. Table 7.7 suggests that multi-

Table 7.6
Distribution of Long-Term Effects, by Age Group

	Under 65	65 and Over	Total
Population (millions)	244.8	37.3	282.1
Utilization Measures (millions)			
Inpatient Stays	−3.2	−3.9	−7.1
Inpatient Nights	−18.6	−30.6	−49.2
Hosp Outpatient + ER Visits	−8.8	−3.7	−12.5
Office Visits	−63.2	−54.8	−118.0
Expenditures ($billions)			
Hospital	−$31.8	−$39.9	−$71.7
Physician	−11.7	−11.4	−23.1
Rx	−16.2	−13.4	−29.6
Other	−4.4	−9.9	−14.3
Total	−$64.1	−$74.6	−$138.7
Days Affected (millions)			
Schooldays Lost	−1.6	0.0	−1.6
Workdays Lost	—39.4	−2.5	−41.9
Total Days Abed	−132.1	−125.1	−257.3
Mortality (thousands)			
Deaths	−119.4	−280.4	−399.8

NOTE: Detail may not add to total due to rounding.

Table 7.7
Long-Term Effects on Prevalences of a 60-Percent Reduction in Odds of Target Conditions

Condition	Baseline	Reduced Incidence	Delta	Percentage Saved
Diabetes	11,511,685	3,465,764	−8,045,921	−69.9%
Chronic Renal Failure	76,387	8,057	−68,330	−89.5%
Lower Limb Involvement	2,710,997	866,105	−1,844,891	−68.1%
Retinopathy	1,213,855	426,868	−786,987	−64.8%
Neuropathy	2,100,691	753,012	−1,347,679	−64.2%
Hypertension	31,524,749	12,986,286	−18,538,463	−58.8%
Hyperlipidemia	11,266,798	3,480,893	−7,785,905	−69.1%
Coronary Artery Disease	3,931,157	959,964	−2,971,192	−75.6%
Cerebrovascular Disease/Stroke	2,811,760	804,811	−2,006,949	−71.4%
Heart Failure	1,428,086	337,946	−1,090,140	−76.3%
Other Heart Disease	16,744,752	5,982,520	−10,762,232	−64.3%
COPD	1,938,975	646,005	−1,292,970	−66.7%
Smoking-Related Cancers	590,213	235,407	−354,806	−60.1%

Table 7.8
Economic Costs of Selected Conditions, from CDC (2003)

Cause	Direct Healthcare Expenditures	Lost Productivity	Total
Cardiovascular Disease/Stroke	$209B	$143B	$352B
Diabetes	$92B	$40B	$132B
Smoking-Related Illness	$75B	$80B	$155B

SOURCE: CDC (2003).

plying the CDC numbers by two-thirds (2/3) would be reasonable. The appropriate comparison, then, is (1) our estimate of $139 billion inflated by 32 percent (i.e., $183 billion), versus (2) the total of the CDC numbers ($376 billion) adjusted for double-counting (leaving $300 billion, let us suppose) and reduced by a factor of 2/3, giving $200 billion—awfully good agreement.

Next, we compared our estimate of the mortality effect with other estimates. The CDC (2004a) published Table 7.9, which suggests that eliminating the chronic conditions included in the table would reduce mortality by two-thirds, or 1,600,000 deaths per year.

This number is four times as large as the reduction of 400,000 that we estimated, but again some adjustments are in order. First, the baseline total we found from the MEPS is 2 million deaths, somewhat lower than the 2.4 million total deaths reported by CDC. It is reasonable to inflate the MEPS numbers by 20 percent to make the baseline totals match. Second, the CDC includes somewhat more cancers than we did. We included only a subset of cancers (see Table 7.1). The National Center for Health Statistics (NCHS) breaks out deaths by cause in greater detail (NCHS GMWK, n.d.), and it appears that the smoking-related cancers we have included account for 179,000 of the 554,000 cancer deaths in Table 7.9.

Moreover, the effects in Table 7.5 correspond to a substantial reduction in the prevalence of our target chronic conditions, but not to their total elimination. Table 7.7 suggests that multiplying the CDC numbers by about 2/3 would be appropriate. The revised comparison, then, is (1) our estimate of 400,000 inflated by 20 percent (i.e., 480,000) or (2) the CDC estimate with the cancer deaths reduced to 179,000 and the results multiplied by 2/3 (i.e., 825,000). This is not close agreement, and suggests to us that the MEPS provides only rough "order of magnitude" estimates of the effects of interventions on mortality.

Table 7.9
Deaths Due to Five Leading Chronic-Disease Killers as a Percentage of All Deaths, United States, 2001

Cause	Number	Percentage
Five leading chronic disease killers	1,611,833	66.7
Diseases of the heart	700,142	29.0
All cancers	553,768	22.9
Stroke	163,538	6.8
Chronic lower respiratory disease	123,013	5.1
Diabetes	71,372	3.0
Other	804,592	33.3
Total	2,416,425	100.0

SOURCE: CDC (2004a).

Aligning and Projecting Effects of a Lifestyle-Change Program

In Chapter Three, we found that utilization and expenditure measures in the MEPS need to be adjusted so that they will be aligned with more-authoritative sources. In addition, to project the effects of these programs from the year 2000 into future years, we must adjust them for demographic changes and further inflate expenditures. Table 7.10 shows the results of these calculations.

The first column repeats the "Total" column from Table 7.6. The second column aligns the utilization measures with the more-authoritative National Hospital Ambulatory Medical Care Survey (NHAMCS), and the expenditures with the more-authoritative NHE, as described in Chapter Three. For subsequent columns, we estimated effects for future years by the same methods as for the first column, but using the person-weights for future years (see Chapter Two) rather than for the year 2000. Then, we adjusted utilization and expenditures to align them with the more-authoritative sources and inflated the expenditures from 2000 to each of the future years, using the escalation factors from Table 3.23.

It may be worthwhile to review just what question Table 7.10 answers. The question is: "Suppose we were able to observe two versions of history. In one, from 1980 onward, everybody adopted the combination of lifestyle changes and (as necessary) medication use that best promotes good health. In the other, from 1980 onward, people continued the lifestyles they have now. What difference would data

Table 7.10
Aligned and Projected Effects of the Lifestyle-Change Program
(assuming 100-percent participation)

Year	Raw MEPS 2000	MEPS Aligned with Authoritative Sources				
		2000	2005	2010	2015	2020
Population (millions)	282.1	282.1	293.3	304.2	315.1	326.1
Utilization Measures (millions)						
Inpatient Stays	−7.1	−7.1	−7.7	−8.3	−9.1	−9.9
Inpatient Nights	−49.2	−49.2	−53.0	−57.5	−63.3	−69.7
Hosp Outpatient + ER Visits	−12.5	−23.1	−25.6	−28.0	−30.0	−31.9
Office Visits	−118.0	−118.0	−127.3	−137.9	−150.3	−163.2
Expenditures ($billions)						
Hospital	−$71.7	−$86.7	−$125.2	−$172.5	−$232.6	−$313.0
Physician	−$23.1	−$35.6	−$51.7	−$74.4	−$104.5	−$146.9
Rx	−$29.6	−$29.6	−$58.2	−$101.0	−$161.6	−$257.4
Other	−$14.3	−$14.3	−$20.8	−$30.6	−$44.6	−$65.7
Total	−$138.7	−$166.2	−$255.9	−$378.5	−$543.3	−$783.0
Days Affected (millions)						
Schooldays Lost	−1.6	−1.6	−1.7	−1.8	−1.8	−1.8
Workdays Lost	−41.9	−41.9	−45.1	−47.3	−48.0	−48.0
Total Days Abed	−257.3	−257.3	−278.7	−299.3	−322.6	−350.4
Mortality (thousands)						
Deaths	−399.8	−399.8	−420.8	−445.0	−488.3	−551.3

collected in the years 2000, 2005, 2010, 2015, and 2020 show between the two versions of history?" The first column is our answer to this question for data from the MEPS of the year 2000. The subsequent columns contain our answers for utilization data from the Nationwide Inpatient Sample (NIS), National Ambulatory Medical Care Survey (NAMCS), and NHAMCS, for expenditures from the NHE, and for health outcomes from the MEPS.

We shift our perspective from the MEPS to the other, provider-based data sources because they are generally considered to be more accurate. We project results into the future because, even if people adopted these lifestyle changes today, it would take many years to realize the full effects. But having made both of these adjustments, we learn little that we could not see from the unadjusted MEPS-based estimates from the year 2000. Utilization and outcomes grow in future years as the population grows and ages. Expenditures grow in response to both population changes and inflation. Our estimates of the long-term effects of lifestyle changes grow in proportion.

Combining Disease-Management and Lifestyle-Change Programs and Adjusting for Lower Participation Rates

Here, we give a simple approximation of the overall effects of combining the program of lifestyle change with the four disease-management programs analyzed in Chapter Six. We also present a method for adjusting the combined results for participation rates that are lower than the 100 percent that we have assumed so far.

Clearly, because the lifestyle changes will have reduced the number of people with chronic conditions, society would not realize the benefits of disease management calculated in Chapter Six. Table 7.7 shows the eligible populations before and after the effects of lifestyle change. To estimate the combined effects, we simply multiply all the effects on utilization, expenditures, and outcomes of each disease management program from Chapter Six by the ratio of the "after" to "before" populations. Then, we add the results to the long-term effects of the lifestyle-change program from Table 7.6. If we assume 100-percent participation in both the lifestyle program and the disease management program, the total dollars saved becomes $147.1 billion per year. Simply adding the savings from disease management would have given a total of $167.2 billion per year.

We can also adjust the numbers to account for reduced participation rates. We assume that the decision to participate in the lifestyle-change program is independent of the decision to participate in a disease management program, so that

P_L = participation rate in the lifestyle program L
P_k = participation rate in disease management program k
ρ_k = ratio of "reduced incidence" to "baseline" population from Table 7.7, for disease management program k.

Then the multipliers of full-participation effects of the various programs are as follows:

$$P_L \qquad \text{for lifestyle program } L \text{ effects}$$
$$[(1 - P_L) \bullet P_k + P_L \bullet P_k \bullet \rho_k] \qquad \text{for disease management program } k \text{ effects.}$$

Table 7.11 applies these formulas for various combinations of participation rates. The formulas have also been implemented in an Excel file, CombineImpacts.xls, that can be accessed at http://www.rand.org/publications/MG/MG408 or on the CD included with printed copies of this monograph. Taking Case E as an example, if only 20 percent of the population participates in the lifestyle

Table 7.11
Combined Effects of Disease Management and Lifestyle Change for Various Participation Rates

	Case A	Case B	Case C	Case D	Case E
Participation Rates (percentage)					
Disease Management	100%	80%	80%	50%	50%
Lifestyle Change	100%	50%	20%	50%	20%
Utilization Measures (millions)					
Inpatient Stays	−8.4	−5.5	−4.0	−4.8	−3.0
Inpatient Nights	−57.8	−38.6	−28.1	−33.3	−21.2
Hosp Outpatient + ER Visits	−14.7	−9.1	−6.0	−8.0	−4.7
Office Visits	−102.9	−39.7	0.1	−46.9	−8.8
Expenditures ($billions)					
Hospital	−$81.2	−$51.7	−$35.1	−$45.8	−$27.3
Physician	−$23.2	−$11.6	−$4.6	−$11.6	−$4.6
Rx	−$28.2	−$13.5	−$4.5	−$14.0	−$5.0
Other	−$14.3	−$7.2	−$2.9	−$7.2	−$2.9
Total	−$146.9	−$83.9	−$47.1	−$78.5	−$39.9
Days Affected (millions)					
Schooldays Lost	−13.1	−10.6	−10.4	−6.9	−6.6
Workdays Lost	−59.2	−39.1	−29.2	−32.3	−21.4
Total Days Abed	−366.5	−270.2	−225.5	−217.1	−160.2
Mortality (thousands)					
Deaths	−516.1	−404.0	−350.8	−327.5	−249.2

program and 50 percent of the eligible population participates in each of the four disease-management programs (diabetes, CHF, asthma, and COPD), we estimate the total savings to be $39.9 billion per year.

CHAPTER EIGHT

The Patient's Role in Disease Management and Lifestyle Changes

James H. Bigelow, Ph.D.

Introduction

Chapter Six assumed that, with the appropriate education and support, chronically ill patients could manage their own chronic conditions effectively. Chapter Seven assumed that everybody could be persuaded to adopt the combination of lifestyle changes and (as necessary) medication use that best promotes good health. That is, everybody refrained from smoking, watched their weight, ate a healthy diet, and exercised. In this chapter, we consider whether most people could be persuaded to adopt healthy habits, and what role Health Information Technology (HIT) could play in making it happen.

In our view, making it happen requires that patients (or consumers, since a person need not be sick to receive health care) adopt a much more active role in their own healthcare than they have done traditionally. Healthcare ceases to be a commodity that healthcare providers deliver. Instead, it becomes an activity in which consumers and providers engage jointly and cooperatively. Think of the analogy of a coach and a player. The coach provides technical knowledge, advice, support, and encouragement to the player. But, ultimately, the player is the one who scores the points. Similarly, when it comes to managing chronic diseases and making lifestyle changes to promote and maintain health, the health care provider has the technical knowledge, but the patient is largely responsible for applying it.

This notion of patient-centeredness differs from the description given in *Crossing the Quality Chasm* (IOM, 2001), which lists six dimensions of patient-centered care:

- Respect for patients' values, preferences, and expressed needs
- Coordination and integration of care
- Information, communication, and education
- Physical comfort

- Emotional support—relieving fear and anxiety
- Involvement of family and friends.

Our notion of patient-centeredness and the notion in the Institute of Medicine (IOM) report intersect at "coordination and integration of care" and "information, communication, and education." The other four dimensions in the IOM report seem related more to patient satisfaction than to patient health. Although we agree that satisfaction with healthcare is important, it is beyond the scope of this study.

Our notion of patient-centeredness goes beyond the IOM notion in seeing the patient as providing his or her own care—the player on the field—rather than as merely participating meaningfully in the decision of what will be done for him or her. For much *acute* care, the IOM notion is appropriate. But for much *chronic* care and many lifestyle choices, the patient is the only person in a position to provide the care. If the patient doesn't do it, it won't get done.

A provocative story by Gawande (2004) involving care for cystic fibrosis (CF) suggests the importance of consumer participation:

> . . . our system for CF care is far more sophisticated than for most diseases. The hundred and seventeen CF centers across the country are all ultra-specialized, undergo a rigorous certification process, and have lots of experience caring for people with CF. They all follow the same guidelines for CF treatment. They all participate in research trials to figure out new and better treatments. You would think, therefore, that their results would be much the same. Yet the differences are enormous.

Expected life span is one of the differences to which he refers. The average CF patient lives to the age of 30. Patients at the best center can expect to live to their mid-40s.

As we interpret Gawande's story, the cause of this difference seems to be that, at the best center, the doctor probes his or her patients searchingly when their test results show even a small decline, persuading, cajoling, and browbeating them—whatever is necessary to discover how the patient is falling short of full, energetic participation in his or her treatment. And then the doctor gets the patient back on track. At the average center, the doctors do not probe nearly as deeply. Small deteriorations in test results are accepted. The doctor may only learn that the patient is skipping his or her treatments when the deterioration in test results becomes large and it may be impossible to reverse the deterioration.

Gawande's story makes the unspoken assumption that if we want the average center to perform as well as the best center, then the average center must change. But perhaps this view is too limited. Perhaps we should consider the CF centers to be only part of a system of care that also includes the patients. With the patient come circumstances and routines and competing demands on his or her time, energy, and attention. If we broaden our view of the system in this way, then we can think of ways to improve overall system performance other than just changing the treatment centers. Perhaps we can make patients full partners in their own healthcare.

In the remainder of this chapter, we first discuss present-day patient adherence with recommendations from healthcare providers. We then review the potential benefits, discussed in previous chapters, of improving patient adherence. Next, we discuss how patient adherence can be improved, first to disease-management programs and then to lifestyle-change programs. We close with a discussion of how much success such efforts to increase adherence might meet.

Present-Day Patient Behavior

There is a considerable body of literature that addresses questions of patient adherence.[1] The World Health Organization (WHO, 2003) offers this definition of *adherence*: "the extent to which a person's behavior—taking medications, following a diet, and/or executing lifestyle changes—corresponds with agreed recommendations from a health care provider."

Experience shows that patients adhere to medication regimes about 50 percent of the time, on average, although there is a great deal of variation from one study to another. Patients adhere to their physicians' lifestyle recommendations only about 10 percent of the time. Adherence over the short term (the first few weeks after the physician's recommendation) is higher, but it declines over time (Roter et al., 1998; Haynes, McDonald, and Garg, 2002).

The United States Preventive Services Task Force (USPSTF) makes recommendations in three categories (chemoprevention, screening, and counseling)[2] concerning what preventive services the primary care physician should provide. Of the three categories, counseling depends particularly strongly for its effectiveness on whether the patient and the provider play their roles.[3] When the USPSTF considers whether to recommend counseling patients on a topic (e.g., tobacco use, diet, or weight loss), it examines the evidence on whether providers have been able to persuade a useful fraction of their patients to act on their counsel.

Interestingly, the USPSTF finds that there is insufficient evidence to determine whether counseling patients in primary care settings to promote physical activity

---

[1] The earliest investigators used the term *compliance,* but recent investigators have objected because the term suggests that the physician is the boss and patients should obey the physician's orders. Investigators now substitute the term *adherence* in order to suggest a more central role for the patient in deciding what advice is to be complied with or adhered to.

[2] See Chapter Five for our examination of selected chemoprevention and screening services.

[3] Patients have a role in chemoprevention and screening, too, but it is much smaller.

leads to sustained increases in physical activity among adult patients. Hence, they do not recommend for or against such counseling, even though there is no question that regular physical activity has proven and substantial health benefits.

There is evidence that people adopt healthier behaviors when they understand the reasons and they have the incentive. For example, the antismoking campaign reduced the fraction of people over 18 that smokes, from 42 percent in 1965 to 23 percent in 2001 (NCHS, 2003)—a 45-percent reduction. It has done so, in part, by making smoking more expensive and, in part, by making it less acceptable. Twenty years ago, almost nobody objected to smokers lighting up in their homes or offices. Today, almost nobody—in California, at least—would fail to object. Other public health successes include the following:[4]

- The fraction of people over 65 not receiving annual influenza vaccinations dropped from 69 percent in 1989 to 37 percent in 2001.
- The fraction of women over 40 who fail to get a mammogram every two years dropped from 71 percent in 1987 to 30 percent in 2000.
- The fraction of women over 18 who fail to get a *Papanicolaou* (PAP) smear at least every three years dropped from 26 percent in 1987 to 19 percent in 2000.

However, the fraction of adults 20–74 years old who are obese has risen, from 13 percent in 1960–1962 to 31 percent in 1999–2000 (NCHS, 2003),[5] which proves that people can adopt unhealthy habits just as easily as healthy ones. Excess weight is a risk factor for many serious (and expensive) medical conditions, including hypertension, heart diseases, diabetes, arthritis-related disabilities, and some cancers. So we are currently seeing a campaign against obesity. California has largely banished junk food from its public schools. Subway® (the chain of sandwich places) advertises its low-fat chicken sandwich, contrasting it with McDonald's™ high-fat Chicken McNuggets™.

Potential Benefits

Our models suggest that potential savings from disease management (Chapter Six) and lifestyle changes (Chapter Seven) could be as large as $147 billion, but only with 100-percent participation by the population. Other potential benefits include 8.4

---

[4] We express these successes in terms of the fraction of people not following recommended health practices, since those are the people who must change their behavior.

[5] The criterion for being overweight is having a body mass index (BMI) of 25 kg/m^2 or more. Being obese is having a BMI of 30 kg/m^2 or more. Thus, the obese group is included in the overweight group. BMI is weight in kilograms divided by the square of height in meters.

million fewer hospital stays (a 30-percent reduction), 13 million fewer schooldays and 59 million fewer workdays lost to sickness (reductions of 7 percent and 9 percent, respectively), and as many as 500,000 deaths postponed (25 percent of total deaths).[6]

Lack of compliance is said to raise healthcare utilization and expenditures, and to increase morbidity and mortality. The Task Force for Compliance (1994) estimated that nonadherence with medications alone costs $100 billion per year, half in increased healthcare expenditures and half in lost productivity. The Life Clinic website[7] claims that nonadherence causes 125,000 potentially preventable deaths, 23 to 40 percent of all nursing home admissions, and 10 percent of hospital admissions.

What Can Be Done?

We discuss disease management separately from promotion of a healthy lifestyle. If a patient has a chronic condition that makes her eligible for disease management, there will be substantial involvement in her case by a healthcare provider or team of providers. By contrast, promoting healthy lifestyle choices for somebody who is basically well should require much less provider involvement. Of the two, effective disease management requires less of a departure from traditional healthcare.

Adherence in a Disease Management Program

As in Chapter Six, we consider disease management programs that are run by primary care providers. The best-studied model for a disease management program is Dr. Wagner's Chronic Care Model (CCM). Bodenheimer, Wagner, and Grumbach (2002a, b) describe the six elements of the CCM:

1. The provider organization has linkages with community resources and policies, so it can arrange for patients to receive services that it does not itself provide.
2. The healthcare organization element encompasses the "structure, goals, and values of a provider organization and its relationships with purchasers, insurers, and other providers [that] form the foundation upon which the remaining 4 components of the chronic care model rest."
3. The CCM offers patients self-management support. The CCM sees the chronically ill patient as the principal caregiver, and self-management support "involves collaboratively helping patients and their families acquire the skills

---

[6] This value counts postponed deaths from both the lifestyle changes and the disease management programs, both estimated from the MEPS.

[7] See http://www.lifeclinic.com/focus/blood/supply_aids.asp; accessed November 26, 2004.

and confidence to manage their chronic illness, providing self-management tools (e.g., blood pressure cuffs, glucometers, diets, and referrals to community resources), and routinely assessing problems and accomplishments."

4. Under the CCM, "the structure of medical practice must be altered, creating practice teams with a clear division of labor and separating acute care from the planned management of chronic conditions. Physicians treat patients with acute problems, intervene in stubbornly difficult chronic cases, and train team members. Non-physician personnel are trained to support patient self-management, arrange for routine periodic tasks, and ensure appropriate follow-up. Planned visits are an important feature of practice redesign."

5. Decision support requires that evidence-based clinical practice guidelines, which provide standards for optimal chronic care, be integrated into daily practice through reminders.

6. The CCM requires Health Information Technology (HIT). "Computerized information has 3 important roles: (1) as reminder systems that help primary care teams comply with practice guidelines; (2) as feedback to physicians, showing how each is performing on chronic illness measures; and (3) as registries for planning individual patient care and conducting population-based care."

Of these elements, the first, third, fourth, and fifth bear most directly on patient self-care. The first element makes information on community resources available to the patient. The third provides education on the nature of the chronic condition and training in how to manage it. The fourth specifies from whom the patient will seek advice and support most of the time. The fifth, guidelines, provides the template for the patient's care plan.

We see HIT as serving more functions than element 6 mentions. It seems clear that HIT should play a role in patient self-management support. If the patient is to be his own principal caregiver, he needs to embrace a plan of care. Developing the plan, and later executing it, requires communication between patient and provider. Communication by email has several advantages over the telephone. The doctor has the question in advance of having to answer it, and he or she can have the relevant documents at hand when replying. Also, there is no need to play "telephone tag." Email messages are written and read at a time convenient for each party. And email can include attachments, such as pictures (even animations), flowcharts, or pamphlets explaining diseases or medications. Finally, email provides a lasting record.

There are several ways in which HIT can help the patient follow his or her care plan. First, HIT can "nag" the patient. Under *nagging,* we include providing reminders, reinforcing knowledge, and cheerleading. For example, Health Hero Network[8] provides a two-way communication device (the Health Buddy) that supports disease management of patients with chronic conditions (e.g., congestive heart failure [CHF] or diabetes). Each day, a short questionnaire is downloaded from the disease management team to the Health Buddy, asking the patient about symptoms, probing the patient's knowledge about his or her medications (What's the water pill for, and why do you think you need it?) and dietary restrictions. The provider can use the information obtained to revise the patient's treatment regime (e.g., adjust medications) in a timely fashion and address any weak areas in the patient's knowledge and understanding. Health Buddy can serve as a communication channel for supplementary education and for messages encouraging the patient to "hang in there, you're doing fine."

HIT can also provide ready access to background information.[9] Background information can take the mystery out of diseases and therapies, and help the patient feel more in control of his life. A generation of first-time mothers obtained similar benefits from Dr. Spock's book *Baby and Child Care*.

It is inefficient for a physician to provide all of the HIT functionality described above. A substantial portion of HIT's contribution to disease management would be more efficiently provided by a communitywide infrastructure. There is no reason that each primary care physician should have to develop his own directory of community resources. Individual providers need not duplicate the service offered by Health Hero Network. Cerner Corporation partnered with Hiawatha Broadband Communications to create Winona Health Online, a communitywide network in Winona, Minnesota, that connects providers and patients. Although it was not specifically focused on chronic illness, over a period of several years the chronically ill have become its heaviest users and most fervent supporters.[10]

Adherence to a Healthy Lifestyle

In many ways, helping people develop healthy habits and manage silent conditions (e.g., hypertension, high cholesterol, and diabetes without complications) is similar to helping people manage a chronic illness that threatens to flare up at any time. Most of the described elements of the CCM have their counterparts in this other arena. These two tasks differ, however, in that the payoff per consumer is much

---

[8] See http://www.healthhero.com; last accessed on July 25, 2005.

[9] For example, see http://www.webMD.com; last accessed July 25, 2005. A source for advice on chronic illness and risk factors (including lifestyle choices) is the National Center for Chronic Disease Prevention and Health Promotion website at http://www.cdc.gov/nccdphp; last accessed July 25, 2005.

[10] Personal communication from Mr. John Larsen, Cerner Corporation, September 17, 2004.

smaller for adopting healthy habits than for managing chronic conditions.[11] In addition, the payoff is generally delayed, and people tend to discount future events.

This observation has two implications. First, a program to foster healthy lifestyle choices should be designed to cost less per participant than a disease management program. Second, it should devote more attention to motivating participants.

Taking up motivation first, we know that consumers give many reasons for not adopting healthy habits. For example, Marge may not believe she needs the blood-pressure-reduction therapy. Hypertension is a largely asymptomatic condition, and Marge feels fine. Hence, she decides taking those pills is unnecessary. Robert may not believe he can follow the advice he is given. Stopping smoking and losing weight are two things people often say they cannot do. George may do a sort of "cost-benefit" analysis, and decide the risk, discomfort, or inconvenience of adopting healthy habits outweighs the potential benefits. Thus, George may decide that he cannot spare the time to exercise, or that exercise leaves him sore.

It is necessary to address each of these issues. The answer to Marge is that uncontrolled hypertension can kill you. If Marge responds to logic and evidence, she might be swayed by estimates of the reduction in her 10-year likelihood of heart attack or stroke. If she does not respond to logic, emotional appeals may work. It is likely, however, that Marge will need constant reinforcement, including a way to see that her efforts are making a difference.

The answer to Robert is a combination of education (other people have done it, and here's how), trial and error, and a step-by-step approach (don't try to quit cold turkey; ration your cigarettes and cut down gradually). There is a difference between "learning about" something (e.g., that to lose weight one must eat less) and "learning to do" it. Even if Robert succeeds for a while, he may not be confident that he can keep it up. He, too, will need constant reinforcement, including visible measures of progress.

George may be persuaded by a combination of the answers to Marge and Robert. Convincing him that exercise will cut his chance of a heart attack will raise his estimate of the benefit, and helping him fit the exercise into his routine will lower his estimate of the cost. Perhaps the combination will "tip" George over the edge. But like the others, George will probably need constant reinforcement.

This need for constant reinforcement stems from the fact that we are creatures of habit. Habits take the place of real-time decisionmaking (i.e., habit determines what you have for breakfast when you don't want to think about it). Learning consciously that she should stop smoking may lead Sally to skip the next cigarette. But until she no longer reaches for a cigarette "without thinking about it," she's still a

---

[11] Chapters Six and Seven suggest that the total payoff from healthy lifestyle choices is the larger of the two. But there are potentially more people eligible for lifestyle improvement than there are eligible for chronic disease management. So the per-participant payoff from healthy lifestyle choices is the smaller of the two.

smoker. Developing new habits or exorcising old ones requires nagging—another name for constant reinforcement.

The only motivation we explicitly mention above is that adopting healthy behaviors will lead to better health outcomes. The participant reduces his chance of a heart attack or stroke. But money can motivate, as well. For example, health insurance premiums could be reduced for members who control their weight or blood pressure (nonsmoking drivers pay less for auto insurance, after all). Or employers could offer prizes for healthy behavior. In addition, people may learn to avoid a behavior if it carries a stigma. In California, smoking has been stigmatized to some degree since the 1994 passage of the smoking ban in workplaces, and it is plausible that this stigmatization is a factor in the long-term decline in smoking that has occurred.

In general, then, a program to help a consumer adopt healthier behaviors and to manage silent conditions should

- tell the participant what his or her risky behaviors are
- estimate the risks those behaviors pose
- work with the participant to develop a strategy for changing those behaviors
- provide the participant with the knowledge and tools to monitor progress
- constantly reinforce the participant's efforts.

The strategy should be customized to the circumstances of the individual participant. For example, it should take advantage of any community resources available to the participant, and take into account any activity limitations or other factors (e.g., allergies) that might affect what the participant could reasonably do.

After motivation comes cost. We now discuss how such a program might be made less costly per participant than the CCM. In Chapter Six, we estimated the cost of a disease management program to be several hundred dollars per participant per year, and most of that money will buy the time of healthcare providers. To reduce the cost, then, we must reduce the need for healthcare providers' time or, for that matter, the time of any personnel.

Use of HIT can lower costs. Indeed, in Chapter Six we estimated that extensive use of HIT in disease management could lower costs by 30 to 50 percent—not enough of a savings for the present purpose. To keep the cost of our lifestyle-improvement program affordable, we must automate some steps, perform some functions on a mass basis, and, perhaps, get some of the work done for free.

Public-service announcements and health educational campaigns are examples of functions provided on a mass basis. Other functions include assembling directories of community resources, preparing templates for strategies that people might follow to change risky behaviors (for example, see the American Heart Association's Just

Move tool[12]) and calculators for estimating health risks from personal characteristics (for example, for calculating the 10-year risk of having a heart attack[13]).

Resources such as these could be incorporated into online services to inventory a person's behaviors, estimate his risks, and develop a strategy for changing the risky behaviors (although it would be wise to have somebody knowledgeable look the strategy over before putting it into practice).

Monitoring progress will be mostly a do-it-yourself process. Each person will measure and record key health indicators, such as blood pressure, cholesterol, or weight. (At present, there is no tool for monitoring cholesterol at home, but surely one could be developed.) The American Heart Association's Just Move tool offers an exercise diary to help the user track his or her progress. Interpreting the results could be as simple as comparing them to a target or as complicated as estimating probabilities of bad outcomes.

One might be able to get some of the work done for free by leveraging community resources, including self-help groups. It seems unlikely that people will adhere to a program of lifestyle modification without the support of other people. In disease management programs, a patient can call the care team for encouragement. A lifestyle-modification program cannot afford a care team. Perhaps community programs and self-help groups can substitute in this role.

The Potential Success Rate

We can only speculate about how many people might be "adherers" five, 10, or 15 years from now. But we speculate that success rates of 50 percent are possible, even for lifestyle changes such as exercising, dieting, quitting smoking, and losing weight. As mentioned above, Haynes, McDonald, and Garg (2002) suggest that current compliance rates with prescriptions for lifestyle change could be as low as 10 percent. On the other hand, the public health examples mentioned earlier show up to 80 percent of the population conforming to recommended behaviors.

Almost every patient gives one or two specific reasons for not adhering, and just about every reason is addressed by at least one intervention. Some consumers may simply be giving excuses: They would not exercise, whatever the doctor says. But for the most part, we take consumers' answers at face value. That is, we accept that each person sees specific barriers to adherence; remove those barriers, address the person's concerns, and he or she will adhere.

---

[12] This tool, a website that includes exercise diaries and educational information, is designed to help you "get the most out of your workouts this year. . . ." Available at http://www.justmove.org; accessed on January 27, 2005.

[13] See http://hin.nhlbi.nih.gov/atpiii/calculator.asp; accessed on January 27, 2005.

Success of 100 percent should not be expected. Some social and cultural reasons for nonadherence may be practically impossible to overcome. Patients may not adhere to medical advice because of their beliefs about the nature of illness (such as the mind-over-matter beliefs of Christian Science). Unstable living conditions (such as those experienced by the homeless) can make adherence difficult.

Poorly educated individuals tend to adhere less to their physician's advice. Goldman and Smith (2002) found that more-educated human immunodeficiency virus (HIV)-positive patients are more likely to adhere to therapy, and that this adherence made them experience improvements in their self-reported general health. Similarly, among diabetics, the less-educated were more likely to switch from one treatment to another, which led to a worsening of general health.

Some people may believe that it's the doctor's job, not theirs, to keep them well. Older adults, especially, might cling to such attitudes. But most of those in the next generation could be persuaded to form healthier habits and attitudes from the beginning. Over time—by which we mean many years—it should be possible to persuade a growing fraction of people to join the ranks of the "adherers." Educational and public health campaigns may make it so.

Although we see reasons to think HIT can help make consumers their own best caregivers, we do not think it will happen quickly or easily. We know of no existing HIT systems that have achieved such a result rapidly. At present, we can only speculate about how that result could be accomplished. To succeed, therefore, people will need to try different approaches, assess them, and improve them—the usual way to learn anything new. It will take many years, and there will be many false steps along the way. But, over time, we think a large fraction of the population can be persuaded to embrace healthy lifestyles.

CHAPTER NINE
Realizing the Potential

James H. Bigelow, Ph.D.

In the preceding chapters, we have estimated the potential benefits of several interventions. By *potential* we mean the maximum effect that could be achieved, assuming that everything goes as well as it possibly could. But, of course the realization will fall short of this ideal. Not all hospitals or physicians will learn to use Health Information Technology (HIT) as effectively as the best. Not all of the chronically ill will learn to manage their conditions at peak effectiveness. Not all consumers will adopt healthy lifestyles. The benefits actually realized will be less than the potential benefits we have estimated, and perhaps much less.

(In passing, we mention that there are factors whose influence is in the other direction. We have estimated the benefits of a relatively small number of specific interventions; there are others that we have not considered. In addition, we have omitted long-term-care spending. A more comprehensive analysis would have yielded larger potential benefits. But realizing the additional potential benefits would be just as problematic as realizing the ones we did estimate.)

As described in Scoville et al. (2005), HIT is an *enabler*: It makes it possible for providers, payers, and consumers to work in more-efficient and -effective ways. But unless providers, payers, and consumers actually change, the benefits will not be realized. Indeed, we defined our interventions in terms of changes in the way the healthcare system works and not in terms of the HIT capabilities that enable those changes to occur.

The literature reports many HIT projects that have failed to achieve their potential, and even successful projects change significantly from initial conception to the eventual working installation. For example, in early 2003 Cedars-Sinai Medical Center in Los Angeles suspended the use of its Patient Care Expert Program (an Electronic Medical Record [EMR]) when doctors complained that it was too hard to use, took too long to enter orders, and its use sometimes resulted in errors (Ornstein, 2003). Difficulty of use and high initial physician time costs are frequently cited as barriers to adoption of HIT (Miller and Sim, 2004). Koppel et al. (2005) have documented errors associated with the use of Computerized Physician Order Entry (CPOE) in a hospital. Failures or setbacks of HIT projects are often blamed on poor software design (as in the Cedars-Sinai case) or on the difficulties of interfacing a new system with legacy systems (McDonald, 1997), but often the problems are, in reality, mismatches between the way work is actually done and the assumptions built into the HIT system about the way work is done (Berg, 1999; Massaro, 1993).

Thus, all HIT projects require some changes in the healthcare organizations in which they are installed. However, most existing HIT applications operate within a single provider organization and require only that the staff of that organization change. Here, we identify two more-drastic, far-reaching changes required by some of our interventions.

One change would coordinate providers in different organizations more closely. The healthcare system is currently fragmented into many independent and uncoordinated hospitals, physician groups, pharmacies, and other provider organizations. The healthcare system is just beginning to experiment with applications that link multiple provider organizations.

The other type of change would make the consumer into an expert provider of his or her own care, rather than a passive recipient. This is the change discussed in Chapter Eight. There, we point out that the consumer is already an active participant but that the healthcare system rarely helps the consumer to participate expertly.

Our interventions, their potential benefits, and the relative risk of realizing that potential are summarized in Table 9.1. The relative risk is our own subjective assessment of how difficult it is likely to be to realize a large fraction of the potential benefit. It is based partly on how many providers have published experiences with the intervention and the strength of the evidence that the intervention works and, partly, on the amount of change required of the healthcare system.

Table 9.1
Summary Potential Net Benefits of Interventions

Class of Intervention	Monetary Net Benefits ($billions)	Relative Health Benefits	Relative Risk
CPOE, inpatient	$1.1	Modest	Low
United States Preventive Services Task Force (USPSTF)-recommended preventive services	Break-even or small net cost	Modest	Medium
CPOE, ambulatory	$31.2	Modest	Medium
Disease management with 100% participation (diabetes, congestive heart failure [CHF], asthma, and chronic obstructive pulmonary disease [COPD])	$28.3	Large	High
Lifestyle change with 100% participation	$138.7	Very large	Very High

Using CPOE to reduce inpatient adverse drug events (ADEs) has the smallest potential benefits, but it has the strongest supporting evidence. In Chapter Four, we assumed inpatient ADE reductions that had actually been achieved, albeit in only a few hospitals. Achieving that potential requires that other hospitals do as well. Moreover, an inpatient EMR can be installed in a single hospital. The hospital provides its own ancillary services, such as pharmacy, laboratory facilities, and radiology department. The physicians initiating orders and the departments fulfilling those orders are under the same organizational roof. There is no need to link multiple providers to the same HIT system. Accordingly, inpatient EMR requires relatively little change from the healthcare system, and we give it a "low" relative risk score.

We have solid evidence of the effectiveness of preventive measures (Chapter Five); the uncertainty concerns how high the participation rate by eligible consumers can be driven. We suppose that a HIT system to promote these services would provide timely reminders to physicians about which of their patients were due for which services, and it would remind patients as well. This system would require more of a connection between physician and patient than is usual at present, so its relative risk score is "medium."

There is less experience with ambulatory ADE reduction and other benefits of ambulatory CPOE than there is with inpatient CPOE; accordingly, we should be less sure about how much of the potential we can actually achieve. Moreover, while an ambulatory EMR installed in a hospital outpatient department can be linked automatically to the hospital departments that provide ancillary services, an EMR in a freestanding clinic or physicians' group must be linked to other independent providers. (Indeed, the literature on ambulatory EMRs mostly describes EMRs installed in hospital outpatient departments.) Few if any physicians' groups provide their own ancillary services in-house. Thus, we award this class of intervention a relative risk score of "medium."

The evidence for disease management benefits consists of a large number of studies, with substantial variation in the details of the intervention and in the population targeted. Accordingly, our estimates of potential benefits have substantial uncertainties. In addition, disease management requires both coordination of multiple providers and expert participation by the patient—i.e., changes to the healthcare system of both kinds. On the other hand, the patient has an immediate incentive to learn how to manage his symptoms. Patients do not, after all, go to the ER for the pleasure and excitement it affords. We assign a relative risk score of "high."

Finally, we have good evidence that if people were to adopt healthier lifestyles, the incidence of many costly diseases would decline, although there is considerable uncertainty concerning just how much the incidences could decline. Moreover, the literature provides no guidance for how to design and implement HIT systems that promote lifestyle change. A program to promote lifestyle change depends even more than disease management on making the patient his or her own expert caregiver, and this is a truly profound change for healthcare. Accordingly, we assign a relative risk score of "very high."

For each of our interventions, there is some risk that the potential benefits will not be fully realized. And, as we move down the rows of Table 9.1, the risk becomes greater. But we need not leave the matter entirely to chance. Taylor et al. (2005) discuss policies that we think could speed adoption of HIT; facilitate the development of the networks needed to connect and coordinate payers, providers, and consumers; and promote efforts to monitor adherence to prevention and disease management guidelines, and measure and improve healthcare quality. Monitoring and measurement are important for all our interventions, but especially so for programs to promote lifestyle change. Because we know least about how to do these tasks, they will require the greatest amount of experimentation before we get them right.

Bibliography

ACS. See American Cancer Society.

Agency for Healthcare Research and Quality (AHRQ), *Clinical Classification Software (CCS) for ICD-9-CM*. Part of the Healthcare Cost and Utilization Project (HCUP). Data and software for aggregating ICD-9 codes to clinical classification codes are available online at http://www.hcup-us.ahrq.gov/toolssoftware/ccs/ccs.jsp (as of February 24, 2005).

Agency for Healthcare Research and Quality (AHRQ), *Medical Expenditure Panel Survey (MEPS)*. Multiple years of data and documentation are available online at http://www.meps.ahrq.gov (as of February 24, 2005).

Agency for Healthcare Research and Quality (AHRQ), *Nationwide Inpatient Sample (NIS)*. Part of the Healthcare Cost and Utilization Project (HCUP). Documentation is available online at http://www.hcup-us.ahrq.gov/nisoverview.jsp (as of February 24, 2005). Data must be purchased.

AHA. See American Hospital Association.

AHRQ. See Agency for Healthcare Research and quality.

Allen, R. M., M. P. Jones, and B. Oldenburg, "Randomised Trial of an Asthma Self-Management Programme for Adults," *Thorax*, Vol. 50, 1995, pp. 731–738.

AMA. See American Medical Association.

American Cancer Society (ACS), *Breast Cancer Facts and Figures 2003–2004*, Atlanta, Ga., 2003a. Available online at http://www.cancer.org (as of January 3, 2005).

American Cancer Society (ACS), *Cancer Facts and Figures 2003*, Atlanta, Ga., 2003b. Available online at http://www.cancer.org (as of January 3, 2005).

American Cancer Society (ACS), *Cancer Facts and Figures 2004*, Atlanta, Ga., 2004. Available online at http://www.cancer.org/docroot/STT/stt_0.asp (as of January 3, 2005).

American Hospital Association (AHA), *AHA Annual Survey Database*. The survey has been conducted since 1946. Data can be ordered from www.ahaonlinestore.com (as of February 24, 2005). Data must be purchased.

American Medical Association (AMA), *Physician Socioeconomic Statistics, 2000–2002 Edition*, Chicago, Ill.: Center for Health Policy Research, 2003.

Aubert, R. E., W. H. Herman, J. Waters, W. Moore, D. Sutton, B. L. Peterson, et al., "Nurse Case Management to Improve Glycemic Control in Diabetic Patients in a Health Maintenance Organization," *Annals of Internal Medicine,* Vol. 129, 1998, pp. 605–612.

Balas, E. A., S. Weingarten, C. T. Garb, D. Blumenthal, S. A. Boren, and G. D. Brown, "Improving Preventive Care by Prompting Physicians," *Archives of Internal Medicine,* Vol. 160, 2000, pp. 301–308.

Bates, D. W., D. J. Cullen, N. Laird, L. A. Peterson, S. D. Small, D. Servi, et al., "Incidence of Adverse Drug Events and Potential Adverse Drug Events," *JAMA,* Vol. 274, No. 1, 1995, pp. 29–34.

Bates, D. W., L. L. Leape, D. J. Cullen, N. Laird, L. A. Petersen, J. M. Teich, et al., "Effect of Computerized Order Entry and a Team Intervention on Prevention of Serious Medication Errors," *JAMA,* Vol. 280, No. 15, 1998, pp. 1311–1316.

Bates, D. W., E. B. Miller, D. J. Cullen, L. Burdick, L. Williams, N. Laird, et al., "Patient Risk Factors for Adverse Drug Events in Hospitalized Patients," *Archives of Internal Medicine,* Vol. 159, 1999, pp. 2553–2560.

Bates, D. W., N. Speil, D. J. Cullen, E. Burdick, N. Laird, L. A. Petersen, et al., "The Costs of Adverse Drug Events in Hospitalized Patients," *JAMA,* Vol. 277, No. 4, 1997, pp. 307–311.

Bates, D. W., J. M. Teich, J. Lee, D. Seger, G. J. Kuperman, N. Ma'Luf, et al., "The Impact of Computerized Physician Order Entry on Medication Error Prevention," *JAMIA,* Vol. 6, No. 4, 1999, pp. 313–321.

Bedell, S. E., S. Jabbour, R. Goldberg, H. Glaser, S. Gobble, Y. Young-Xu, T. B. Graboys, and S. Ravid, "Discrepancies in the Use of Medications: Their Extent and Predictors in an Outpatient Practice," *Archives of Internal Medicine,* Vol. 160, 2000, pp. 2129–2134.

Berg, A. O., and J. D. Allen, "Introducing the New U.S. Preventive Services Task Force," *American Journal of Preventive Medicine,* Vol. 20 (Suppl 3), 2001, pp. 3–4. Available online at http://www.ahrq.gov/clinic/uspstfix.htm (as of July 17, 2003).

Berg, M., "Patient Care Information Systems and Health Care Work: A Sociotechnical Approach," *International Journal of Medical Informatics,* Vol. 55, 1999, pp. 87–101.

Berger, J., J. Slezak, N. Stine, et al., "Economic Impact of a Diabetes Disease Management Program in a Self-Insured Health Plan: Early Results," *Disease Management,* Vol. 4, 2001, pp. 65–74.

Bernstein, A. B., E. Hing, A. J. Moss, K. F. Allen, A. B. Siller, and R. B. Tiggle, *Health Care in America: Trends in Utilization,* Hyattsville, Md.: National Center for Health Statistics, 2003. Available online at http://www.cdc.gov/nchs/data/misc/healthcare.pdf (as of February 7, 2005).

Birkmeyer, J. D., C. M. Birkmeyer, D. E. Wennberg, and M. Young, *Leapfrog Patient Safety Standards. The Potential Benefits of Universal Adoption,* Washington, D.C.: Academy Health, The Leapfrog Group, 2000. Available online at http://www.leapfroggroup.org (as of April 12, 2001).

Birkmeyer, J. D., C. M. Birkmeyer, D. E. Wennberg, and M. Young, *Leapfrog Patient Safety Standards. Economic Implications,* Washington, D.C.: Academy Health, The Leapfrog Group, 2001. Available online at http://www.leapfroggroup.org (as of April 12, 2001).

Bodenheimer, T., E. H. Wagner, and K. Grumbach, "Improving Primary Care for Patients with Chronic Illness," *JAMA,* Vol. 288, No. 14, 2002a, pp. 1775–1779.

Bodenheimer, T., E. H. Wagner, and K. Grumbach, "Improving Primary Care for Patients with Chronic Illness: The Chronic Care Model, Part 2," *JAMA,* Vol. 288, No. 15, 2002b, pp. 1909–1914.

Bolton, M. B., B. C. Tilley, J. Kuder, T. Reeves, and L. R. Schultz, "The Cost and Effectiveness of an Education Program for Adults Who Have Asthma," *Journal of General Internal Medicine,* Vol. 6, 1991, pp. 401–407.

Bott, U., S. Bott, D. Hemmann, and M. Berger, "Evaluation of a Holistic Treatment and Teaching Programme for Patients with Type 1 Diabetes Who Failed to Achieve Their Therapeutic Goals Under Intensified Insulin Therapy," *Diabetic Medicine,* Vol. 17, No. 9, 2000, pp. 635–643.

Bourbeau, J., M. Julien, F. Maltais, M. Rouleau, A. Beaupré, R. Bégin, et al., "Reduction of Hospital Utilization in Patients with Chronic Obstructive Pulmonary Disease," *Archives of Internal Medicine,* Vol. 163, 2003, pp. 585–591.

Bower, Anthony G., *The Diffusion and Value of Healthcare Information Technology,* Santa Monica, Calif.: RAND Corporation, MG-272-HLTH, 2005.

Bridges, C. B., W. W. Thompson, M. I. Meltzer, G. R. Reeve, W. J. Talamonti, N. J. Cox, et al., "Effectiveness and Cost-Benefit of Influenza Vaccination of Healthy Working Adults: A Randomized Controlled Trial," *JAMA,* Vol. 284, No. 13, 2000, pp. 1655–1663.

Bronner, L. L., D. S. Kanter, and J. E. Manson, "Primary Prevention of Stroke," *New England Journal of Medicine,* Vol. 333, No. 21, 1995, pp. 1392–1400.

Brown, A., "Heart Failure," in E. A. Kerr, S. M. Asch, E. G. Hamilton, and E. A. McGlynn, eds., *Quality of Care for Cardiopulmonary Conditions: A Review of the Literature and Quality Indicators,* Santa Monica, Calif.: RAND, MR-1282-AHRQ, 2000.

Burton, W. N., C. M. Connerty, A. B. Schultz, C. Y. Chen, and D. W. Edington, "Bank One's Work Site–Based Asthma Disease Management Program," *Journal of Occupational and Environmental Medicine,* Vol. 43, 2001, pp. 75–82.

CDC. See Centers for Disease Control and Prevention.

CDC Diabetes Cost-Effectiveness Study Group, "Cost-Effectiveness of Intensive Glycemic Control, Intensified Hypertension Control, and Serum Cholesterol Level Reduction for Type 2 Diabetes," *JAMA,* Vol. 287, No. 19, 2002, pp. 2542–2551.

Center for the Advancement of Health (CFAH), *Selected Evidence for Behavioral Approaches to Chronic Disease Management in Clinical Settings: Asthma,* Washington, D.C., 2000. Available online at http://www.cfah.org (as of March 4, 2004).

Centers for Disease Control and Prevention (CDC), *The Burden of Chronic Diseases and Their Risk Factors: National and State Perspectives, 2004,* Atlanta, Ga.: Centers for Disease Control and Prevention, February 2004a. Available online at http://www.cdc.gov/nccdphp/burdenbook2004/index.htm (as of November 5, 2004).

Centers for Disease Control and Prevention (CDC), *The Burden of Chronic Diseases and Their Risk Factors 2004,* Atlanta, Ga.: National Center for Chronic Disease Prevention and Health Promotion, 2004b. Available online at http://www.cdc.gov/nccdphp (as of November 5, 2004).

Centers for Disease Control and Prevention (CDC), *The Burden of Chronic Diseases and Their Risk Factors: National and State Perspectives, 2002,* Atlanta, Georgia, February 2002. Available online at http://www.cdc.gov/nccdphp/burdenbook2002/index.htm (as of January 28, 2004).

Centers for Disease Control and Prevention (CDC), *The Power of Prevention,* Atlanta, Georgia: National Center for Chronic Disease Prevention and Health Promotion, 2003. Available online at http://www.cdc.gov/nccdphp (as of November 5, 2004).

Centers for Disease Control and Prevention, National Center for Health Statistics, Hyattsville, Md., mortfinal2001_workorig290f.pdf, 2003. Available online at http://www.cdc.gov/nchs/datawh/statab/unpubd/mortabs.htm (last accessed August 3, 2005).

Centers for Disease Control and Prevention (CDC), "Prevention and Control of Influenza: Recommendations of the Advisory Committee on Immunization Practices (ACIP)," *Morbidity and Mortality Weekly Report,* April 14, 2000. Available online at http://www.cdc.gov/epo/mmwr/preview/mmwrhtml/rr4903a1.htm (as of November 11, 2004).

Centers for Disease Control and Prevention (CDC), "Prevention of Pneumococcal Disease: Recommendations of the Advisory Committee on Immunization Practices (ACIP)," *Morbidity and Mortality Weekly Report,* April 4, 1997. Available online at http://www.cdc.gov/epo/mmwr/preview/mmwrhtml/00047135.htm (as of November 11, 2004).

Centers for Medicare and Medicaid Services (CMS), *Health Accounts,* Baltimore, Md., 2001. Available online at http://www.cms.hhs.gov/statistics/nhe/definitions-sources-methods/dsm.pdf (as of February 27, 2004).

Centers for Medicare and Medicaid Services (CMS), *Health Accounts,* Baltimore, Md. Available online at http://www.cms.hhs.gov/statistics/nhe/default.asp (as of February 27, 2004).

Centers for Medicare and Medicaid Services (CMS), *Healthcare Cost Reporting Information System (HCRIS),* Baltimore, Md. Described at http://www.cms.hhs.gov/data/cost_reports/default.asp (as of February 18, 2005). Data may be purchased.

Centers for Medicare and Medicaid Services (CMS), *Payment Allowances for the Influenza Virus Vaccine (CPT 90658) and the Pneumococcal Vaccine (CPT 90732) When Payment Is Based on 95 Percent of the Average Wholesale Price (AWP),* Washington, D.C., Pub 100-20

One-Time Notification, September 17, 2004. Available online at http://www.cms.hhs.gov/medlearn/refimmu.asp (as of December 29, 2004).

CFAH. See Center for the Advancement of Health.

Chan, D. S., C. W. Callahan, and C. Moreno, "Multidisciplinary Education and Management Program for Children with Asthma," *American Journal of Health System Pharmacy*, Vol. 58, No. 15, 2001, pp. 1413–1417.

Chiasson, J. L., R. G. Josse, R. Gomis, M. Hanefeld, A. Karasik, and M. Laakso, "Acarbose Treatment and the Risk of Cardiovascular Disease and Hypertension in Patients with Impaired Glucose Tolerance: The STOP-NIDDM Trial," *JAMA*, Vol. 290, No. 4, 2003, pp. 486–494.

Clark, C. M., Jr., and D. A. Lee, "Prevention and Treatment of the Complications of Diabetes Mellitus," *New England Journal of Medicine*, Vol. 332, No. 18, 1995, pp. 1210–1217.

Clarke, J. L., and D. B. Nash, "The Effectiveness of Heart Failure Disease Management: Initial Findings from a Comprehensive Program," *Disease Management*, Vol. 5, No. 4, 2002, pp. 215–223.

Classen, D. C., S. L. Pestotnik, R. S. Evans, J. F. Lloyd, and J. P. Burke, "Adverse Drug Events in Hospitalized Patients: Excess Length of Stay, Extra Costs, and Attributable Mortality," *JAMA*, Vol. 277, No. 4, 1997, pp. 301–306.

Cline, C. M., B. Y. Israelsson, R. B. Willenheimer, K. Broms, and L. R. Erhardt, "Cost Effective Management Programme for Heart Failure Reduces Hospitalization," *Heart*, Vol. 80, 1998, pp. 442–446.

CMS. See Centers for Medicare and Medicaid Services.

Corrigan, J. M., and M. Donaldson, eds., *To Err Is Human: Building a Safer Health System*, Washington, D.C.: National Academy Press, 1999.

Cox, B. G., and R. Iachan, "A Comparison of Household and Provider Reports of Medical Conditions," *Journal of the American Statistical Association*, Vol. 82, No. 400, 1987, pp. 1013–1018.

Demakis, J. G., C. Beauchamp, W. L. Cull, R. Denwood, S. A. Eisen, R. Lofgren, et al., *JAMA*, Vol. 184, No. 11, 2000, pp. 1411–1416.

Diabetes Control and Complications Trial Research Group, "The Effect of Intensive Treatment of Diabetes on the Development and Progression of Long-Term Complications in Insulin-Dependent Diabetes Mellitus," *New England Journal of Medicine*, Vol. 329, No. 14, 1993, pp. 977–986.

Diabetes Prevention Research Group, "Reduction in the Incidence of Type 2 Diabetes with Lifestyle Intervention or Metformin," *New England Journal of Medicine*, Vol. 346, No. 6, 2002, pp. 393–403.

Domurat, E. S., "Diabetes Managed Care and Clinical Outcomes: The Harbor City, California, Kaiser Permanente Diabetes Care System," *American Journal of Managed Care*, Vol. 5, 1999, pp. 1299–1307.

Earnshaw, S. R., A. Richter, S. W. Sorensen, T. J. Hoerger, K. A. Hicks, M. Engelgau, et al., "Optimal Allocation of Resources Across Four Interventions for Type 2 Diabetes," *Medical Decision Making,* Vol. 22, No. 5 (Suppl), 2002, pp. S80–S91.

Edwards, W. S., D. M. Winn, V. Kurlantzick, S. Sheridan, M. L. Berk, S. Retchin, and J. G. Collins, "Evaluation of National Health Interview Survey Diagnostic Reporting," *Vital and Health Statistics Report,* Series 2, No. 120, 1994. Available online at http://www.cdc.gov/nchs/products/pubs/pubd/series/ser.htm (as of January 28, 2004).

Eliaszadeh, P., H. Yarmohammade, H. Nawaz, J. Boukhalil, and D. Katz, "2001: Congestive Heart Failure Case Management: A Fiscal Analysis," *Disease Management,* Vol. 4, 2001, pp. 25–32.

Erickson, P., R. Wilson, and I. Shannon, "Years of Healthy Life," Atlanta, Ga.: Centers for Disease Control, Statistical Note No. 7, 1995. Available online at http://www.cdc.gov/nchs/data/statnt/statnt07.pdf (as of February 19, 2003).

Gallefoss, F., and P. S. Bakke, "Impact of Patient Education and Self-Management on Morbidity in Asthmatics and Patients with Chronic Obstructive Pulmonary Disease," *Respiratory Medicine,* Vol. 94, No. 3, 2000, pp. 279–287.

Gallefoss, F., and P. S. Bakke, "Cost-Benefit and Cost-Effectiveness Analysis of Self-Management in Patients with COPD—A 1-Year Follow-Up Randomized, Controlled Trial," *Respiratory Medicine,* Vol. 96, No. 6, 2002, pp. 424–431.

Gawande, A., "The Bell Curve: What Happens When Patients Find Out How Good Their Doctors Really Are?" *The New Yorker,* December 6, 2004.

Gibson, P. G., H. Powell, J. Coughlan, A. J. Wilson, M. Abramson, P. Haywood, et al., "Self-Management Education and Regular Practitioner Review for Adults with Asthma," *Cochrane Database System Review,* Vol. 1, 2003, p. CD001117.

Gillespie, J., "The Value of Disease Management—Part 1: Balancing Cost and Quality in the Treatment of Congestive Heart Failure: A Review of Disease Management Services for the Treatment of Congestive Heart Failure," *Disease Management,* Vol. 4, No. 2, 2001, pp. 41–51.

Gillespie, J., "The Value of Disease Management—Part 3: Balancing Cost and Quality in the Treatment of Asthma." *Disease Management,* Vol. 5, No. 4, 2002, pp. 225–232.

Girosi, Federico, Robin Meili, and Richard Scoville, *Extrapolating Evidence of Health Information Technology Savings and Costs,* Santa Monica, Calif.: RAND Corporation, MG-410-HLTH, 2005. Available online at http://www.rand.org/publications/MG/MG410 as of September 14, 2005.

Glassman, P. A., personal communication, December 9, 2003.

Glassman, P. A., B. Simon, P. Belperio, and A. Lanto, "Improving Recognition of Drug Interactions: Benefits and Barriers to Using Automated Drug Alerts," *Medical Care,* Vol. 40, No. 12, 2002, pp. 1161–1171.

GOLD, *Global Initiative for Chronic Obstructive Lung Disease (GOLD). Executive Summary,* 2004. Online at www.goldcopd.com (as of January 25, 2005).

Goldman, D. P., and J. P. Smith, "Can Patient Self-Management Help Explain the SES Health Gradient?" *Proceedings of the National Academy of Sciences,* Vol. 99, No. 16, 2002, pp. 10929–10934. Available online at http://www.pnas.org (as of May 29, 2003).

Hadley, J., and J. Holahan, "Covering the Uninsured: How Much Would It Cost?" *Health Affairs,* Web Exclusive, Vol. W3, 2003, pp. 250–265.

Hammer, M., and J. Champy, *Reengineering the Corporation: A Manifesto for Business Revolution,* New York: HarperBusiness, 1993.

Haynes, R. B., H. P. McDonald, and A. X. Garg, "Helping Patients Follow Prescribed Treatment: Clinical Applications," *JAMA,* Vol. 288, No. 22, 2002, pp. 2880–2883.

Heffler, S., S. Smith, S. Keehan, M. K. Clemens, M. Zezza, and C. Truffer, "Health Spending Projections Through 2013," *Health Affairs,* Web Exclusive, Vol. W4, 2004, pp. 79–93.

Hillestad, R., J. Bigelow, A. Bower, F. Girosi, R. Meili, R. Scoville, and R. Taylor, "Can Electronic Medical Record Systems Transform Healthcare? An Assessment of Potential Health Benefits, Savings, and Costs," *Health Affairs,* Vol. 24, No. 5, September 14, 2005.

Hoerger, T. J., R. Harris, K. A. Hicks, K. Donahue, S. Sorensen, and M. Engelgau, "Screening for Type 2 Diabetes Mellitus: A Cost-Effectiveness Analysis," *Annals of Internal Medicine,* Vol. 140, No. 9, 2004, pp. 689–699 (Technical appendix, pp. E700–E710).

Homer, J., G. Hirsch, M. Minniti, and M. Pierson, "Models for Collaboration: How System Dynamics Helped a Community Organize Cost-Effective Care for Chronic Illness," Presentation to Institute for Healthcare Improvement, Pursuing Perfection Partners meeting, April 28, 2003.

Hunter, M. H., and D. E. King, "COPD: Management of Acute Exacerbations and Chronic Stable Disease," *American Family Physician,* Vol. 64, No. 4, 2001, pp. 603–612.

Institute of Medicine (IOM), *Crossing the Quality Chasm: A New Health System for the 21st Century,* Washington, D.C.: National Academy Press, 2001.

IOM. See Institute of Medicine.

Jessup, M., and S. Brozena, "Heart Failure," *New England Journal of Medicine,* Vol. 348, No. 20, 2003, pp. 2007–2018.

Jha, A. K., G. J. Kuperman, E. Rittenberg, J. M. Teich, and D. W. Bates, "Identifying Hospital Admissions Due to Adverse Drug Events Using a Computer-Based Monitor," *Pharmacoepidemiology and Drug Safety,* Vol. 10, No. 2, 2001, pp. 113–119.

Johnson, A. E., and M. E. Sanchez, "Household and Medical Provider Reports on Medical Conditions: National Medical Expenditure Survey, 1987," *Journal of Economic and Social Measures,* Vol. 19, 1993, pp. 199–223.

Johnson, J. A., and J. L. Bootman, "Drug-Related Morbidity and Mortality," *Archives of Internal Medicine,* Vol. 155, 1995, pp. 1949–1956.

Johnston, D., E. Pan, J. Walker, D. W. Bates, and B. Middleton, *The Value of Computerized Provider Order Entry in Ambulatory Settings,* Wellesley, Mass.: Center for Information Technology Leadership, 2003. Available for purchase at http://www.citl.org (as of February 23, 2005).

Johnston, D., E. Pan, J. Walker, D. W. Bates, and B. Middleton, *Patient Safety in the Physician's Office: Assessing the Value of Ambulatory CPOE,* Wellesley, Mass.: Center for Information Technology Leadership, 2004. Prepared for the California HealthCare Foundation. Available online at http://www.chcf.org (as of April 12, 2004).

Jowers, J. R., A. L. Schwartz, and D. G. Tinkelman, "Disease Management Program Improves Asthma Outcomes," *American Journal of Managed Care,* Vol. 6, No. 5, 2000, pp. 585–589.

Kauppinen, R., V. Vilkka, H. Sintonen, T. Klaukka, and H. Tukiainen, "Long-Term Economic Evaluation of Intensive Patient Education During the First Treatment Year in Newly Diagnosed Adult Asthma," *Respiratory Medicine,* Vol. 95, No. 1, 2001, pp. 56–63.

Kelly, C. S., S. W. Shield, M. A. Gowen, N. Jaganjac, C. L. Andersen, and G. L. Strope, "Outcomes Analysis of a Summer Asthma Camp," *Journal of Asthma,* Vol. 35, 1998, pp. 165–171.

Kerlikowske, K., P. Salzmann, K. Phillips, J. A. Cauley, and S. R. Cummings, "Continuing Screening Mammography in Women Aged 70 to 79 Years: Impact on Life Expectancy and Cost-Effectiveness," *JAMA,* Vol. 282, No. 22, 1999, pp. 2156–2163.

Kerr, E. A., S. M. Asch, E. G. Hamilton, and E. A. McGlynn, eds., *Quality of Care for Cardiopulmonary Conditions: A Review of the Literature and Quality Indicators,* Santa Monica, Calif.: RAND, MR-1282-AHRQ, 2000.

Knox, D., and L. Mischke, "Implementing a Congestive Heart Failure Disease Management Program to Decrease Length of Stay and Cost," *Journal of Cardiovascular Nursing,* Vol. 14, 1999, pp. 55–74.

Koppel, R., J. P. Metlay, A. Cohen, et al., "Role of Computerized Physician Order Entry Systems in Facilitating Medication Errors," *JAMA,* Vol. 293, No. 10, 2005, pp. 1197-1203.

Kotses, H., I. L. Bernstein, and D. I. Bernstein, "A Self-Management Program for Adult Asthma. Part I: Development and Evaluation," *Journal of Allergy and Clinical Immunology,* Vol. 95, 1995 pp. 529–540.

Kotses, H., C. Stout, K. McConnaughy, J. A. Winder, and T. L. Creer, "Evaluation of Individualized Asthma Self-Management Programs," *Journal of Asthma,* Vol. 33, 1996, pp. 113–118.

Krishna, S., B. D. Francisco, E. A. Balas, P. Konig, G. R. Graff, and R. W. Madsen, "Internet-Enabled Interactive Multimedia Asthma Education Program: A Randomized Trial," *Pediatrics,* Vol. 111, No. 3, 2003, pp. 503–510.

Lahdensuo, A., T. Haahtela, and J. Herrala, "Randomised Comparison of Guided Self-Management and Traditional Treatment of Asthma over One Year," *British Medical Journal,* Vol. 312, 1996, pp. 748–752.

Larsen, J., personal communication, September 17, 2004.

Lazarou, J., B. H. Pomeranz, and P. N. Corey, "Incidence of Adverse Drug Reactions in Hospitalized Patients: A Meta-Analysis of Prospective Studies," *JAMA,* Vol. 279, No. 15, 1998, pp. 1200–1205.

Leape, L. L., D. W. Bates, D. J. Cullen, J. Cooper, H. J. Demonaco, T. Gallivan, R. Hallisey, J. Ives, N. Laird, G. Laffel, R. Nemeskal, L. A. Petersen, K. Porter, D. Servi, B. F. Shea, S. D. Small, B. J. Sweitzer, B. T. Thompson, and M. V. Vliet, "Systems Analysis of Adverse Drug Events," *JAMA,* Vol. 274, 1995, pp. 35–43.

Leape, L. L., A. I. Kabcenell, T. K. Gandhi, P. Carver, T. W. Nolan, and D. M. Berwick, "Reducing Adverse Drug Events: Lessons from a Breakthrough Series Collaborative," *Journal of Quality Improvement,* Vol. 26, No. 6, 2000, pp. 321–331.

Leiberman, D. A., "Management of Chronic Pediatric Diseases with Interactive Health Games: Theory and Research Findings," *Journal of Ambulatory Care Management,* Vol. 24, No. 1, 2001, pp. 26–38.

Lynne, D., "Diabetes Disease Management in Managed Care Organizations," *Disease Management,* Vol. 7, No. 1, 2004, pp. 47–60.

Machlin, S. R., J. W. Cohen, and J. M. Thorpe, "Measuring Inpatient Care Use in the United States: A Comparison Across Five Federal Data Sources," *Journal of Economic and Social Measurement,* Vol. 20, 2000, pp. 141–151.

Machlin, S. R., J. L. Valluzzi, F. M. Chevarley, and J. M. Thorpe, "Measuring Ambulatory Health Care Use in the United States: A Comparison of 1996 Estimates Across Four Federal Surveys," *Journal of Economic and Social Measurement,* Vol. 27, 2001, pp. 57–69.

Maeder, T., "Good Health Is Just a Costly Way to Die," *Red Herring Magazine,* September 19, 2001.

Marle, Mv-Av., Mv. Ballegooijen, GJv. Oortmarssen, R. Boer, and J.D.F. Habbema, "Cost-Effectiveness of Cervical Cancer Screening: Comparison of Screening Policies," *Journal of the National Cancer Institute,* Vol. 94, No. 3, 2002, pp. 193–204.

Massaro, T. A., "Introducing Physician Order Entry at a Major Academic Medical Center: I. Impact on Organizational Culture and Behavior," *Academic Medicine,* Vol. 68, No. 1, 1993, pp. 20–25.

Mayo, P. H., J. Richman, and W. Harris, "Results of a Program to Reduce Admissions for Adult Asthma," *Annals of Internal Medicine,* Vol. 112, 1990, pp. 864–871.

McCulloch, D. K., M. J. Price, M. Hindmarsh, and E. H. Wagner, "A Population-Based Approach to Diabetes Management in a Primary Care Setting: Early Results and Lessons Learned," *Effective Clinical Practice,* Vol. 1, No. 1, 1998, pp. 12–22.

McDonald, C. J., "The Barriers to Electronic Medical Record Systems and How to Overcome Them," *JAMIA,* Vol. 4, No. 3, 1997, pp. 213–221.

McDonald, C. J., S. L. Hui, and W. M. Tierney, "Effects of Computer Reminders for Influenza Vaccination on Morbidity During Influenza Epidemics," *MD Computing*, Vol. 9, No. 5, 1992, pp. 304–312.

McGlynn, E. A., S. M. Asch, J. Adams, J. Keesey, J. Hicks, A. DeCristofaro, and E. A. Kerr, "The Quality of Health Care Delivered to Adults in the United States," *New England Journal of Medicine*, Vol. 348, No. 26, 2003, pp. 2635–2645.

Miller, R. H., and I. Sim, "Physicians' Use of Electronic Medical Records: Barriers and Solutions," *Health Affairs*, Vol. 23, No. 2, 2004, pp. 116–126.

National Center for Health Statistics (NCHS), *Classification of Diseases and Functioning and Disability.* This document provides a description of the ICD-9 codes; it is available online at www.cdc.gov/nchs/icd9.htm (as of February 24, 2005). The Centers for Medicare and Medicaid Services (CMS) oversees all revisions to the clinical modification of the ICD-9 (ICD-9-CM), which we are using. Version 19 of the ICD-9-CM is available online at, www.cms.hhs.gov/providers/pufdownload/default.asp (as of May 6, 2003).

National Center for Health Statistics (NCHS), *GMWK290F: Deaths for 113 Selected Causes by 10-Year Age Group, Race, and Sex: United States, 1999-2001,* Hyattsville, Md., n.d. Available online at http://www.cdc.gov/nchs/datawh/statab/unpubd/mortabs/ gmwk290A_10.htm (as of February 24, 2005).

National Center for Health Statistics (NCHS), *Health, United States, 2003,* Hyattsville, Md. Available online at http://www.cdc.gov/nchs/hus.htm (as of on December 23, 2003).

National Center for Health Statistics, *International Classification of Diseases,* Revision 9, Hyattsville, Md.

National Center for Health Statistics (NCHS), *National Ambulatory Medical Care Survey (NAMCS),* Hyattsville, Md. Multiple years of data and documentation are available online at http://www.cdc.gov/nchs/about/major/ahcd/ahcd1.htm (as of February 24, 2005).

National Center for Health Statistics (NCHS), *National Hospital Ambulatory Medical Care Survey (NHAMCS),* Hyattsville, Md. Multiple years of data and documentation are available online at http://www.cdc.gov/nchs/about/major/ahcd/ahcd1.htm (as of February 24, 2005).

National Center for Health Statistics (NCHS), *National Nursing Home Survey (NNHS),* Hyattsville, Md. Multiple years of data and documentation are available online at http://www.cdc.gov/nchs/about/major/nnhsd/nnhsd.htm (as of February 24, 2005).

National Pharmaceutical Council (NPC), *Disease Management for Asthma,* Reston, Va., August 2004a. Available online at http://www.npcnow.org (as of November 29, 2004).

National Pharmaceutical Council (NPC), *Disease Management for Chronic Obstructive Pulmonary Disease,* Reston, Va., September 2003. Available online at http://www.npcnow.org (as of November 29, 2004).

National Pharmaceutical Council (NPC), *Disease Management for Diabetes,* Reston, Va., February 2004b. Online at http://www.npcnow.org (as of November 29, 2004).

National Pharmaceutical Council (NPC), *Disease Management for Heart Failure,* Reston, Va., October 2004c. Available online at http://www.npcnow.org (as of November 29, 2004).

NCHS. See National Center for Health Statistics.

Needleman, J., P. I. Buerhaus, S. Mattke, M. Stewart, and K. Zelevinsky, *Nurse Staffing and Patient Outcomes in Hospitals,* Cambridge, Mass.: Harvard School of Public Health, Report for the Health Resources Service Administration, 2001. Available online at http://www.bhpr.hrsa.gov/nursing (as of December 29, 2003).

Norris, S. L., P. J. Nichols, C. J. Caspersen, R. E. Glasgow, M. M. Engelgau, L. Jack, et al., "The Effectiveness of Disease and Case Management for People with Diabetes. A Systematic Review," *American Journal of Preventive Medicine,* Vol. 24 (4 Suppl), 2002, pp. 15–38.

NPC. See National Pharmaceutical Council.

Ornstein, C., "Hospital Heeds Doctors, Suspends Use of Software," *Los Angeles Times,* January 23, 2003.

Overhage, J. M., W. M. Tierney, and X-H Zhou, "A Randomized Trial of Corollary Orders to Prevent Errors of Omission," *JAMIA,* Vol. 4, No. 5, 1997, pp. 364–375.

Patel, P. H., C. Welsh, and M. B. Foggs, "Improved Asthma Outcomes Using a Coordinated Care Approach in a Large Medical Group," *Disease Management,* Vol. 7, No. 2, 2004, pp. 102–111.

Peng, C. C., P. A. Glassman, I. R. Marks, C. Fowler, B. Castiglione, and C. B. Good, "Retrospective Drug Utilization Review: Incidence of Clinically Relevant Potential Drug-Drug Interactions in a Large Ambulatory Population," *Journal of Managed Care Pharmacy,* Vol. 9, No. 6, 2003, pp. 513–522.

Peters, A. L., and M. B. Davidson, "Application of a Diabetes Managed Care Program. The Feasibility of Using Nurses and a Computer System to Provide Effective Care," *Diabetes Care,* Vol. 21, No. 7, 1998, pp. 1037–1043.

Pettersson, E., A. Gardulf, G. Nordstrom, C. Svanberg-Johnsson, and G. Bylin, "Evaluation of a Nurse-Run Asthma School," *International Journal of Nursing Studies,* Vol. 36, 1999, pp. 145–151.

Philbin, E. F., T. A. Rocco, N. W. Lindenmuth, K. Ulrich, M. McCall, and P. L. Jenkins, "The Results of a Randomized Trial of a Quality Improvement Intervention in the Care of Patients with Heart Failure," *American Journal of Medicine,* Vol. 109, 2000, pp. 443–449.

Phillips, K. A., M. G. Shlipak, P. Coxson, P. A. Heidenreich, M. G. Hunink, P. A. Goldman, et al., "Health and Economic Benefits of Increased Beta-Blocker Use Following Myocardial Infarction," *JAMA,* Vol. 284, No. 21, 2000, pp. 2748–2754.

Piette, J. D., M. Weinberger, F. B. Kramer, and S. J. McPhee, "Impact of Automated Calls with Nurse Follow-Up on Diabetes Treatment Outcomes in a Department of Veterans

Affairs Health Care System: A Randomized Controlled Trial," *Diabetes Care,* Vol. 24, No. 2, 2001, pp. 2202–2208.

Pignone, M., S. Saha, T. Hoerger, and J. Mandelblatt, *Cost-Effectiveness Analysis of Colorectal Cancer Screening: A Systematic Review for the U.S. Preventive Services Task Force,* Rockville, Md., May 2002. Available online at www.preventiveservices.ahrq.gov (as of July 17, 2003).

Rich, M. W., V. Beckham, C. Wittenberg, C. L. Leven, K. E. Freedland, and R. M. Carney, "A Multidisciplinary Intervention to Prevent the Readmission of Elderly Patients with Congestive Heart Failure," *New England Journal of Medicine,* Vol. 333, 1995, 1190–1195.

Rich-Edwards, J. W., J. E. Manson, C. H. Hennekens, and J. E. Buring, "The Primary Prevention of Coronary Heart Disease in Women," *New England Journal of Medicine,* Vol. 332, No. 26, 1995, pp. 1758–1766.

Ross, S., D. Togger, and D. Desjardins, "Asthma Disease Management Program Cuts Readmissions," *Hospital Case Management,* Vol. 6, No. 10, 1998, pp. 197–200.

Rossiter, L. F., M. Y. Whitehurst-Cook, R. E. Small, et al., "The Impact of Disease Management on Outcomes and Cost of Care: A Study of Low-Income Asthma Patients," *Inquiry,* Vol. 37, No. 2, 2000, pp. 188–202.

Roter, D. L., J. A. Hall, R. Merisca, B. Nordstrom, D. Cretin, and B. Svarstad, "Effectiveness of Interventions to Improve Patient Compliance," *Medical Care,* Vol. 36, No. 8, 1998, pp. 1138–1161.

Rubin, R. J., K. A. Dietrich, and A. D. Hawk, "Clinical and Economic Impact of Implementing a Comprehensive Diabetes Management Program in Managed Care," *Journal of Clinical Endocrinology and Metabolism,* Vol. 83, No. 8, 1998, pp. 2635—2642.

Sadur, C. N., N. Moline, M. Costa, D. Michalik, D. Mendlowitz, S. Roller, et al., "Diabetes Management in a Health Maintenance Organization. Efficacy of Care Management Using Cluster Visits," *Diabetes Care,* Vol. 22, No. 12, 1999, pp. 2011–2017.

Salzmann, P., K. Kerlikowske, and K. Phillips, "Cost-Effectiveness of Extending Screening Mammography Guidelines to Include Women 40 to 49 Years of Age," *Annals of Internal Medicine,* Vol. 127, No. 11, 1997, pp. 955–965.

Scoville, Richard P., Roger Taylor, Robin Meili, and Richard Hillestad, *How HIT Can Help: Process Change and the Benefits of Healthcare Information Technology,* Santa Monica, Calif.: RAND Corporation, TR-270-HLTH, 2005.

Selden, T. M., K. R. Levit, J. W. Cohen, S. H. Zuvekas, J. F. Moeller, D. McKusick, and R. H. Arnett, "Reconciling Medical Expenditure Estimates from the MEPS and the NHA, 1996," *Health Care Financing Review,* Vol. 23, No. 1, 2001, pp. 161–178.

Shah, N. B., E. Der, C. Ruggerio, P. A. Heidenreich, and B. M. Massie, "Prevention of Hospitalizations for Heart Failure with an Interactive Home Monitoring Program," *American Heart Journal,* Vol. 135, 1998, pp. 373–378.

Shea, S., W. DuMouchel, and L. Bahamonde, "A Meta-Analysis of 16 Randomized Controlled Trials to Evaluate Computer-Based Clinical Reminder Systems for Preventive Care in the Ambulatory Setting," *JAMIA,* Vol. 3, No. 6, 1996, pp. 399–409.

Sidorov, J., R. Gabbay, R. Harris, R. D. Shull, S. Girolami, J. Tomcavage, R. Starkey, and R. Hughes, "Disease Management for Diabetes Mellitus: Impact on Hemoglobin A1c," *American Journal of Managed Care,* Vol. 6, No. 11, 2000, pp. 1217–1226.

Sidorov, J., R. Shull, J. Tomcavage, S. Girolami, N. Lawton, and R. Harris, "Does Diabetes Disease Management Save Money and Improve Outcomes? A Report of Simultaneous Short-Term Savings and Quality Improvement Associated with a Health Maintenance Organization–Sponsored Disease Management Program Among Patients Fulfilling Health Employer Data and Information Set Criteria," *Diabetes Care,* Vol. 25, No. 4, 2002, pp. 684–689.

Snyder, J. W., J. Malaskovitz, J. Griego, J Persson, and W. Flatt, "Quality Improvement and Cost Reduction Realized by a Purchaser Through Diabetes Disease Management," *Disease Management,* Vol. 6, No. 4, 2003, pp. 233–241.

Sonnenberg, A., F. Delco, and J. M. Inadomi, "Cost-Effectiveness of Colonoscopy in Screening for Colorectal Cancer," *Annals of Internal Medicine,* Vol. 133, No. 8, 2000, pp. 573–584.

Sonnenberg, F. A., and J. R. Beck, "Markov Models in Medical Decision Making: A Practical Guide," *Medical Decision Making,* Vol. 13, 1993, pp. 322–338.

Steffens, B., "Cost-Effective Management of Type 2 Diabetes: Providing Quality Care in a Cost-Constrained Environment," *American Journal of Managed Care,* Vol. 6 (Suppl), 2000, pp. S697–S703.

Stothard, A., and K. Brewer, "Dramatic Improvement in COPD Patient Care in Nurse-Led Clinic," *Nursing Times,* Vol. 97, No. 24, 2001, pp. 36–37.

Taplin, S. H., W. Barlow, N. Urban, M. T. Mandelson, D. J. Timlin, L. Ichikawa, and P. Nefcy, "Stage, Age, Comorbidity, and Direct Costs of Colon, Prostate, and Breast Cancer Care," *Journal of the National Cancer Institute,* Vol. 87, No. 6, 1995, pp. 417–426.

Taylor, Roger, Anthony Bower, Federico Girosi, James Bigelow, and Richard Hillestad, "Promoting Health Information Technology: A Case for More Aggressive Government Action," *Health Affairs,* Vol. 24, No. 5, September 14, 2005.

The Task Force for Compliance, *Noncompliance with Medications: An Economic Tragedy with Important Implications for Health Care Reform,* Baltimore, Md., 1994, pp. 1–32. Available online at http://www.npcnow.org/resources.asp (as of November 26, 2004).

Tolley, G., D. Kenkel, and R. Fabian, eds., *Valuing Health for Policy,* Chicago, Ill.: The University of Chicago Press, 1994.

U.S. Census Bureau, *1997 Economic Census,* Washington, D.C. Available online at http://www.census.gov/epcd/www/ec97stat.htm (as of February 24, 2005).

U.S. Census Bureau, *National Population Projections: II. Detailed Files,* Washington, D.C. Available online at http://www.census.gov/population/www/projections/natdet.html (as of February 24, 2005).

U.S. Census Bureau, *Service Annual Survey,* Washington, D.C. Available online at http://www.census.gov/econ/www/servmenu.html (as of February 24, 2005).

United States Pharmacopeia (USP), "Top-50 Drug Errors," Rockville, Md. Available online at http://www.usp.org/patientSafety/tools/top50DrugErrors.html (as of December 11, 2003).

United States Preventive Services Task Force (USPSTF), "Adult Immunizations—Including Chemoprophylaxis Against Influenza A," *Guide to Clinical Preventive Services,* 2nd ed., Rockville, Md., 1996, Chapter 66. Available online at http://www.ahrq.gov/clinic/uspstfix.htm (as of December 13, 2004).

United States Preventive Services Task Force (USPSTF) (corresponding author, A. O. Berg), *Screening for Colorectal Cancer: Recommendations and Rationale,* Washington, D.C., AHRQ Pub No. 03-510A, July 2002a. Available online at http://www.ahrq.gov/clinic/uspstfix.htm (as of July 17, 2003).

United States Preventive Services Task Force (USPSTF) (corresponding author, A. O. Berg), *Screening for Breast Cancer: Recommendations and Rationale,* Washington, D.C., AHRQ Pub No. 03-507A, August 2002b. Available online at http://www.ahrq.gov/clinic/uspstfix.htm (as of July 17, 2003).

United States Preventive Services Task Force (USPSTF), *Screening for Cervical Cancer: Recommendations and Rationale* (corresponding author, A. O. Berg), Washington, D.C., AHRQ Pub No. 03-515A, January 2003. Online at http://www.ahrq.gov/clinic/uspstfix.htm (as of July 17, 2003).

USP. See United States Pharmacopeia.

USPSTF. See United States Preventive Services Task Force.

Vaccaro, J., J. Cherry, A. Harper, et al., "Utilization Reduction, Cost Savings and Return on Investment for the Pacificare Chronic Heart Failure Program: Taking Charge of Your Heart Health," *Disease Management,* Vol. 4, 2001, pp. 131–138.

Villagra, V. G., and T. Ahmed, "Effectiveness of a Disease Management Program for Patients with Diabetes," *Health Affairs (Millwood),* Vol. 23, No. 4, 2004, pp. 255–266.

Wagner. E. H., L. C. Grothaus, N. Sandhu, M. S. Galvin, M. McGregor, K. Artz, and E. A. Coleman, "Chronic Care Clinics for Diabetes in Primary Care: A System-Wide Randomized Trial," *Diabetes Care,* Vol. 24, No. 4, 2001, pp. 695–700.

Wang, S. J., B. Middleton, L. A. Prosser, C. G. Bardon, C. D. Spurr, P. J. Carchidi, et al., "A Cost-Benefit Analysis of Electronic Medical Records in Primary Care," *American Journal of Medicine,* Vol. 114, 2003, pp. 397–403.

Weinstein, M. C., P. G. Coxson, L. W. Williams, T. M. Pass, W. B. Stason, and L. Goldman, "Forecasting Coronary Heart Disease Incidence, Mortality, and Cost: The

Coronary Heart Disease Policy Model," *American Journal of Public Health,* Vol. 77, No. 11, 1987, pp. 1417–1426.

Wennberg, J. E., and M. M. Cooper, eds., *The Dartmouth Atlas of Health Care 1999,* Lebanon, N.H.: Dartmouth Medical School, Center for Evaluative Clinical Sciences, 1999. Available online at www.dartmouthatlas.org (as of February 8, 2005).

West, J. A., N. H. Miller, K. M. Parker, D. Senneca, G. Ghandour, M. Clark, et al., "A Comprehensive Management System for Heart Failure Improves Clinical Outcomes and Reduces Medical Resource Utilization," *American Journal of Cardiology,* Vol. 79, 1997, pp. 58–63.

WHO. See World Health Organization.

Wilson, P.W.F., R. D. D'Agostino, B. Levy, A. M. Belanger, H. Silbershatz, and W. B. Kannel, "Prediction of Coronary Heart Disease Using Risk Factor Categories," *Circulation,* Vol. 97, 1998, pp. 1837–1847.

Wilson, S. R., P. Scamagas, D. F. German, et al., "A Controlled Trial of Two Forms of Self-Management Education for Adults with Asthma," *American Journal of Medicine,* Vol. 94, 1993, pp. 564–576.

World Health Organization (WHO), *Adherence to Long-Term Therapies: Evidence for Actions,* Geneva, Switzerland, 2003. Available online at http://www.who.int/chronic_conditions/adherencereport/en/ (as of November 24, 2004).

Yarnell, K.S.H., K. I. Pollak, T. Ostbye, K. M. Krause, and J. L. Michener, "Primary Care: Is There Time Enough for Prevention?" *American Journal of Public Health,* Vol. 93, No. 4, 2003, pp. 635–641.

Yoon, R., D. K. McKenzie, A. Bauman, and D. A. Miles, "Controlled Trial Evaluation of an Asthma Education Programme for Adults," *Thorax,* Vol. 48, 1993, pp. 1110–1116.

Zajac, B., "Measuring Outcomes of a Chronic Obstructive Pulmonary Disease Management Program," *Disease Management,* Vol. 5, 2002, pp. 9–23.

Zeiger, R. S., S. Heller, M. H. Mellon, J. Wald, R. Falkoff, and M. Schatz, "Facilitated Referral to Asthma Specialist Reduces Relapses in Asthma Emergency Room Visits," *Journal of Allergy and Clinical Immunology,* Vol. 87, 1991, pp. 1160–1168.